AROMATHERAPY HANDBOOK

FOR BEAUTY,

HAIR, AND

SKIN CARE

AROMATHERAPY HANDBOOK

FOR BEAUTY,

HAIR, AND

SKIN CARE

ERICH KELLER

Translated into English by
CHRISTINE GRIMM

Healing Arts Press
Rochester, Vermont

Healing Arts Press
One Park Street
Rochester, Vermont 05767
www.InnerTraditions.com

Healing Arts Press is a division of Inner Traditions International

First published in German under the title *Essenzen der Schönheit* by Goldmann Verlag, Munich 1991
First U.S. edition 1992

Note to the reader: This book is intended as an informational guide. The remedies, approaches, and techniques described herein are meant to supplement, and not to be a substitute for, professional medical care or treatment. They should not be used to treat a serious ailment without prior consultation with a qualified healthcare professional.

LIBRARY OF CONGRESS CATALOGING-IN-PUBLICATION DATA
Keller, Erich
    [Essenzen der Schönheit. English]
    Aromatherapy handbook for beauty, hair, and skin care / Erich Keller
       p. cm.
    Translation of : Essenzen der Schönheit.
    Includes bibliographical references and index.
    ISBN 0-89281-433-0; 0-89281-831-X
    1. Aromatherapy. 2. Essences and essential oils. 3. Skin—Care and hygiene. 4. Hair—Care and hygiene. 5. Beauty, Personal. I. Title.
RM666.A68K4413   1991
615'.321—dc20   91-26587
                                                       CIP

Printed and bound in Canada.

10 9 8 7 6 5 4 3 2 1

Text design by Virginia L. Scott

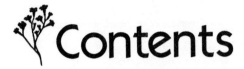# Contents

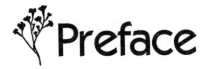# Preface

This book describes the effects of essential oils and their potential use in natural cosmetics and as healing agents in aromatherapy. It contains advice for those who would like to make their own natural cosmetics, those whose professions involve work with natural cosmetics, and those who are simply interested in the subject of natural skin and hair care and who would like to know something about the ingredients used and their effects.

I have worked with essential oils for some years now. In an earlier book, now available in English as *The Complete Home Guide to Aromatherapy*, I described all the information regarding essential oils that was available at that time. It was clear to me that these natural treasures could be used to create products for the gentle and effective care of skin and hair. In fact, most of the questions I subsequently received from readers and students on the topic of aromatherapy concerned the cosmetic use of these oils, and I realized that the subject required a book of its own. From the broad spectrum of standard recipes that are available from books on cosmetics and aromatherapy, I have chosen here a sampling of basic formulas for the safe and easy production at home of creams, lotions, toners, facial and body oils, masks, packs, ointments, shampoos, hair rinses, and the like. The recipes given in these pages have all been tested, and some are even identical to those used by cosmetic manufacturers. In addition, by studying many formulas I have developed a number of new recipes for this book.

Cosmetics with essential oils are holistic, natural products that serve as perfume, beauty aid, and medicine all at the same time. Their task is to take care of the skin, regulate its functions, maintain its health, heal diseases and irritations, stimulate and support the body's own healing powers, and—as the most pleasant result—promote and protect your natural beauty. They are actually easier to make than traditional natural cosmetics since here there is no need to macerate, boil, and filter herbs. The concentrated essential oils can be obtained in small bottles that are ready for immediate use but which can also be stored for a long time without any loss in their effectiveness.

In contrast to synthetic cosmetics, cosmetics prepared with essential oils use natural components only. No chemical dyes, synthetic fragrances, chemical preservatives, or harmful substances are included. The contents are always pure and beneficial to the skin. What is most important, when you make your own cosmetics you are the manufacturer: thus you know precisely what ingredients have been used and in what quantities—a secret that the producers of commercial synthetic cosmetics will never divulge to consumers.

Essential oils, the heart of these cosmetics, have been used for thousands of years by many different cultures. Their effects have long been demonstrated for the most part through the work of naturopathy. They all have one element that cannot be manufactured in a laboratory: vital force. The sap of life and the "soul" of a plant are in these essential oils. They have a gentle and natural effect on the skin, hair, and sense of smell. If you have already dealt with essential oils, then you know about the amazingly subtle effects these fragrances can have on the disposition and on the body.

I wish you the same experience that I have had in the preparation of this book—the pleasure of discovering, creating, and enjoying the products of these fragrant gifts of nature.

1 Cosmetics

History of the Development of Cosmetics

In the twentieth century, the French perfumer and chemist Gattefossé, working in Grasse, examined the healing effects of essential oils after some surprisingly positive experiences with them. He called this field of endeavor "aromatherapy" and published his first book on the topic in 1928. His countryman, the physician Jean Valnet (author of a *Handbook of Aromatherapy*), was inspired by Gattefossé's reports and began to treat his patients exclusively with herbal extracts and essential oils. He and the French biochemist Marguerite Maury, who explored the use of essential oils and skin care and rejuvenating the body, substantiated their claims with medical evidence, thereby supporting and supplementing a tradition of ancient knowledge about the healing and stimulating effects of essential oils.

Following the Second World War, the production of synthetic cosmetics experienced an upswing that has basically continued to the present day. Indeed, decorative cosmetics have become the

1

facial uniform of modern, civilized women throughout the world through the operations of the commercial cosmetic giants, whose products continue to contain extremely harmful substances. The end of the 1960s however, brought signs of a return to a more natural lifestyle. Since that time, advances in the ecology movement and environmental consciousness have led to a more critical view of the substances used in synthetic cosmetics as well as to the emergence of a growing number of small cosmetic manufacturers offering natural cosmetics.

Since the 1980s, companies have been founded in Europe and the United States that exclusively manufacture natural cosmetics. Some of these companies offer products that contain both natural substances and synthetic preservatives, emulsifiers, dyes, foaming agents, and fragrances. Such products are perhaps best referred to as "semi-natural," for they are neither completely natural nor completely "synthetic." (Although many of the major commercial cosmetic firms have also made a practice of adding terms such as "natural" or "organic" to their products, these products in fact have not fundamentally changed.) In the meantime, however, other new companies have begun to offer fresh cosmetics that are free of all synthetic substances. These products are available today in health food stores, natural food stores, herb shops, and natural cosmetic stores, whereas synthetic cosmetics are sold in drugstores, pharmacies, perfumeries, large cosmetic shops and department stores; thus a clear separation has been made between product types—to the advantage of the consumer. Today, essential oils and herbal extracts have again become an elementary component of natural cosmetics, thereby completing a cycle that began thousands of years ago.

Synthetic Cosmetics

A brief comparison of synthetic and natural cosmetics, illustrating the composition and effects of each, should provide a better idea of what to expect from both types of cosmetics.

In the field of synthetic, commercially produced cosmetics, new substances are constantly being developed that claim to be nonirritating and to care for and heal the skin. These products actually do contain effective synthetic substances which are not found naturally in such concentrations, particularly not at the cheap prices made possible by the industrial-chemical production process. Although nature can now be quite convincingly imitated in the laboratory, the vital force that is the essence of organic, natural substances is missing. Synthetic cosmetics cannot be rejected across the board as "inferior" cosmetics; however, there are significant arguments for preferring pure natural cosmetics.

All synthetic cosmetic articles contain preservatives and/or disinfectants that impair or even eliminate the effectiveness of any natural substances they may contain. These agents are foreign substances (e.g., formaldehyde, hexachlorophene, and quarternium-15) that are known to damage the skin's flora and protective "acid mantle." Moreover, they promote aging of the skin by reducing its water-absorbent capacities. As they penetrate the skin's layers, such substances remove the skin's elasticity. The wrinkles resulting from this process are then likely to be treated with some anti-aging cream that is equally likely to contain harmful preservatives.

The dilemma, of course, is that it is not possible to produce cosmetic articles that can last for months or even years without preservatives. In addition, some disinfecting agent is needed since germs can form in the tubes and jars once they have been opened. These circumstances naturally mean that truly natural cosmetics can be produced without such substances only at great effort and correspondingly high costs. But they *are* available!

A view of the commercial production of shampoos (a product that directly influences the scalp) is equally sobering. Here we find aggressive tensides and occasionally strong alkaline soaps that are not beneficial for the skin. The industry likes to add sodium lauryl sulfates or sodium laureth sulfates, substances that foam and clean thoroughly. In fact, they clean so thoroughly that the protective acid mantle and the skin's natural sebum are completely washed away. As a result, the scalp is off balance, and in turn endangers the hair that grows from it. In Germany, consumer research has established that commercial shampoos even contain pain-relieving agents as they themselves can cause pain. Although there is no doubt that preservatives such as formaldehyde and nitrosamines are harmful to the skin, they are still permitted to be used as preservatives in the United States. Add to this picture the combined effects of other ingredients such as chemical thickeners, preservatives, dyes, and fragrances, which may penetrate the hair follicles and thereby enter the bloodstream. One such ingredient, dioxan, a substance that has been widely used in the manufacture of shampoos by the cosmetic industry, is known to be carcinogenic. We may be impressed by a label's list of substances that are beneficial to skin and hair, such as aloe vera, jojoba oil, and herbal extracts. Yet these valuable substances are subsequently rendered ineffective by additives. As long as the product label is not complete, there is no way to be certain that natural substances are present in proportions that allow them to provide their natural effect.

A further example: The popular foaming agents that create beautifully bubbling bath additives, shower gels, shampoos, and toothpastes are irritating to the skin as well. The foam attacks and destroys the skin flora, and the skin becomes even more brittle and dry, as is made apparent by the itching that then must be relieved with a moisturizing lotion or cream.

To compensate for this negative effect the manufacturers of soaps, shampoos, bubble baths, and shower gels now add oils or fats to replace those lost because of the active cleansing substances. The moisture-bonding agents also serve to prevent drying. The critical consumer then asks: why use such aggressive agents in the first place? Because they foam and clean so well, which advertising has suggested for decades is of utmost importance.

The same negative consequences apply to the chemical dyes and fragrances contained in many cosmetic articles. Since chemical cosmetics usually do not have an appealing color and either have no smell or an actually unpleasant one, they must be redesigned to appeal to the nose and eyes of the consumer: hence the addition of further chemicals to mask the base chemicals. Furthermore, the production of an emulsifier from water and oil—the basis of almost all creams, lotions, and shampoos—is possible only with an emulsifying agent or thickener. Because of their cost and perishability, natural emulsifying agents and thickeners are never used. Yet the chemical emulsifying agents that are used instead impair the effectiveness of the natural substances or attack the skin flora.

The problem is even more serious in ornamental cosmetics such as lipsticks. The thin, unprotected skin of the mouth is directly affected by their harmful dyes, which then enter into the metabolism. Similarly, mascaras, eye shadows, and eyeliners contain heavy metals and chemical dyes that penetrate the skin, are stored on a long-term basis in the body, and poison it.

Among the ready-made cosmetics are moisturizing creams and lotions made of water and mineral oils that "provide" the upper layer of the skin with moisture for some hours and then paradoxically cause it to dry out. Anti-wrinkle or anti-aging creams that temporarily cause the surface skin to swell are very popular as well. The skin looks fresh and smooth for several hours, but soon falls back into its old condition. The "wonder drug" substances these creams contain—collagen, elastin, and the like—smooth the skin and give a temporary impression of improvement—until the next time the face is washed. In fact, once the the natural collagen and elastin in the connective tissue has attained an age-appropriate, hardened condition wrinkles cannot be "ironed out." What *is* possible at this juncture is to stimulate the formation of new skin cells and to discourage the further loss of moisture.

Although the cosmetic industry recommends creams with collagen and elastin for wrinkles, it has never been proved that the skin forms new collagen or elastin if these substances are applied externally. Both of these "wonder drugs" appear in two forms: as a substance distilled from animal bones and hooves that absorbs water poorly, and as natural collagen and elastin, derived through extraction from the connective tissue (tendons, cartilage, and skin) of slaughtered animal wastes. These substances represent proteins that are foreign to the body, although they do work to bind moisture in the epithelium and give the creams and lotions their silky character.

Next, a word about vitamin and hormone creams. Clearly it is simpler and more economical for a person to take in vitamins in the form of food and to let the body produce its own hormones, which simply requires healthy and balanced nutrition, and a harmonious lifestyle. (It does seem paradoxical to rub something on the skin that actually belongs in the stomach!)

Studies in Europe have found that the skin can only absorb ten percent of most synthetic creams. This is partly because the mineral oils they contain cannot be dissolved by the skin fats, and partly because the large molecules of the active substances cannot penetrate the upper layer of skin, with a few important exceptions (e.g., liposomes and essential fatty acids). In most instances, ninety percent of the cream "sits" on the skin, does not penetrate, and serves only as protection against the loss of further moisture—an effect that can be achieved more naturally and for less money with a facial oil.

Many cosmetics promising "wondrous" effects have been offered over the past few decades: liposome, vitamins, collagen, elastin, and hormones. Yet the condition of peoples' skin has not improved. The consumer increasingly suffers from eczema, itching and irritations of the skin, dryness, extreme oiliness, and damaged skin flora—symptoms that certainly relate to deteriorating environmental conditions and inadequate nutrition, but that are widely influenced by aggressive, synthetic cleansing and skin care agents.

What of the promise of hypoallergenic products offered by the cosmetic industry? The likelihod of skin irritations resulting from certain substances seems to be ruled out by labels such as "allergy-tested" and "hypoallergenic"—as if any individual consumer's reaction to this or that substance could be determined on a mass scale! Yet "allergy-tested" means only that the product *was* tested, it does not tell us what the results were. Indeed, the very fact that products have to be tested for their tendency to provoke allergies should give cause for concern.

As is widely known, the tests conducted by cosmetics manufacturers are based on animal experiments that take the lives of over one hundred million animals a year. These animals are injected with or forced to ingest substances, or have substances sprayed into their eyes (which are held open with clamps) or applied to their skin.

Yet even the "positive results" obtained by this widespread form of animal torture cannot guarantee cosmetics without side effects, as we now know after decades of uncritically consuming cosmetics and medications. As consumers, we are not told whether the "positive" results of a given test were extremely positive or merely this side of tolerable; and often the long-term effect of some toxic or carcinogenic substance in a cosmetic product is discovered only after many years.

Price is an additional factor to weigh in reviewing the worth of ready-made cosmetics. In view of the low cost of manufacturing synthetic raw materials, it must seem odd that creams cost four times the price of the ingredients for a natural, fresh product. Even the hormones and vitamins whose inclusion is felt to make products more valuable—and worth their high price—can be synthetically manufactured for pennies.

What about labeling? We may be impressed by a listing of beneficial ingredients such as aloe vera, jojoba oil, or herbal extracts. And in fact all of these substances may be contained in the product. But a general listing of ingredients does not tell us how much of each ingredient is included and/or whether it is a natural substance. A label may proclaim that its cream contains rose oil, a highly desirable and costly oil—but the actual ingredient may just as well be a synthetic oil with the identical chemical structure and same smell but without the natural effect of rose oil. Another product may include "jojoba" in its name but actually contain the much cheaper but less effective jojoba flour rather than pure jojoba oil. A label such as "with extract of birch" says nothing about how much birch is actually contained in the product. In short, until adequate labeling of cosmetics is regulated, there is no way to know how much of any one substance is contained in the product, whether the substances are natural, or what kind of actual effect they will have.

Cosmetics Made with Essential Oils

Before we turn to cosmetics with essential oils, let us briefly consider the ingredients of natural cosmetics. Of course the purest substances should be used—but can such expectations be completely fulfilled by any type of cosmetic product today? Pesticides, toxic chemicals, and pollutants which are harmful to health exist everywhere; even if the plants are grown organically, our planet itself is so polluted by now that an absolutely pure raw material as such may no longer exist. Today we can only judge raw materials according to their relative purity.

A second point to consider is the actual availability of the raw materials for natural cosmetics—our natural resources. If every cosmetic article and all industrial fragrances were to be produced from natural substances, our present rate of consumption would soon mark the peppermint in the meadows, the lemons on the trees, lavender blossoms and the sandalwood trees as endangered species. There are simply too many people using too many cosmetics. Deteriorating environmental influences, toxic substances in the air and water, air pollution, and aggressive cleansing and skin care agents, and their negative effects on our skin and hair have all led to an enormous grooming effort, driven by massive advertising for cosmetics. Unfortunately, at the same time many people pay little attention to nutrition, despite the fact that the food available in our latitudes contains all the necessary vitamins and minerals for healthy skin and hair.

Solutions to these problems are dependent upon a change in our consciousness and our behavior in regard to nutrition, grooming, environment, and nature. We should not have to kill off our fauna and flora in order to naturally groom and cleanse ourselves. Cosmetics prepared at home with essential oils require only small amounts of raw materials. Since the skin and hair can recover relatively quickly from chemical treatment when cared for with natural cosmetics, anyone who embarks on such a plan can expect to be freed from the need to keep using numerous and extravagant grooming products. However, all measures for natural care must also be accompanied by a healthy lifestyle. Included in this plan would be foods rich in vitamins and minerals as well as the avoidance of drugs, nicotine, alcohol, caffeine, and stress.

In contrast to commercial ready-made cosmetics, the homemade ones offered in these pages make exclusive use of natural substances. They contain no mineral oils, synthetic substances, synthetic preservatives or dyes. The vegetable oils themselves have excellent skin care qualities, contain nutrients, and regulate moisture.

The essential oils listed here are ideal for skin care since they heal, vitalize the tissue, stimulate the renewal of the cells, cleanse and rejuvenate the skin, promote the metabolism, prevent or soothe irritations and infections, have an antiseptic effect, and guarantee the stability of the cosmetics in a natural way. Essential oils work in a way that is—to one or another degree—antibacterial, bacteriostatic, and fungicidal.

In addition, many essential oils contain plant hormones (phytohormones), and some contain substances similar to estrogen (anise, verbena, fennel, eucalyptus, sage) that affect the skin (collagen) and tissue (tone). These plant hormones are absorbed by the skin and influence the hormonal equilibrium of the body. They have the effect of tautening the skin, rejuvenating (renewing the cells), and regulating sebaceous gland production—an important effect in the treatment of oily skin, oily hair, and acne. Plant hormones do not have the side effects of animal hormones, which could make the skin appear spongy and swollen when used over a longer period of time.

Essential oils also stimulate the endocrine glands and influence the secretion of the body's own hormones. For example, thyme oil has a balancing effect on the adrenal cortex, which produces estrogen. Estrogen regulates the elasticity of the skin and the connective tissue, the muscle tone, and the burning of body fat. Estrogen can improve the condition of the skin and tissue, as can be seen in many women who have taken birth control pills. Thyme oil speeds up the gland secretions of the skin, activates the blood circulation, increases the blood pressure, purifies the skin, and generally has a stimulating effect on the organism. It is used in cases of hair loss, for general hair care, healing of skin and wounds, oral hygiene, and care of the gums, as well as in the treatment of pimples and boils.

Each essential oil will have a number of effects and thus can be used for various symptoms. An oil can also be selected for its scent, since healing and grooming substances should have a good fragrance.

The most important argument for using essential oils in cosmetics has to do with their *vital force* and their *naturalness*. The life within us can best be cared for and healed with living things. We have a strong affinity for plants, particularly the flower oils—their blossoms are the "face" of the plant—that are used for facial care in essential oil cosmetics. When the facial skin is treated with flower oils, it receives the entire stored solar energy and vital force of the essential oil. The flower's oils are easily dissolved by the sebaceous fat, and their molecules are so small that they can actually penetrate the skin to reach the lowest level and even affect the deeper tissue and organs.

Essential oils also act upon mood and various body functions through the sense of smell. The scent of the essential oils used in any preparation influences your spirit and physical well-being. The effect on the sense of smell is especially intense when oils are used to create perfumes or aroma baths. The scent is guaranteed to be stimulating. These effects of the oils make them into holistic treatment and grooming substances.

The application of essential oils for the care and healing of the skin has been proved over thousands of years and is supported by current scientific studies. There are no animal experiments carried out by the manufacturers and dealers to examine the effectiveness of their products. The oils have no side effects when they are used as directed, and are largely free from allergens. If an allergy seems to develop after the oil is used repeatedly, please refer to the description of the essential oil in the second chapter of this book. Still, occasional sensitization should not present serious problems: since a number of oils are suited to each skin type, another oil can easily be substituted. Natural cosmetics with essential oils are gentle, subtle cosmetics. They are not likely to work as quickly as synthetic products, but they work effectively and continually. Your skin may well need some time to adjust to the new natural substances, but its condition will assuredly improve.

The preparation of natural cosmetics is simple, and no machinery is required. In contrast to traditional natural cosmetics, there is no labor-intensive and time-consuming boiling of herbs, no straining, and no filtering. The ingredients are fundamentally the essential oils in small bottles and other natural components such as vegetable oils, lanolin, clay, cocoa butter, beeswax, honey, pure water, and flower water. All equipment can be stored in a small area.

When you make natural cosmetics you will also experience the creative process of doing it yourself. You can change the recipes, play with the ingredients, and at the same time create something valuable for yourself: a product whose effects are clear and whose ingredients are more economical and fresher than anything available at a store. Further, if you should choose or need at any point to buy natural cosmetic products, you will be armed with the best possible background to read labels, ask questions, and reach intelligent consumer decisions.

Handling essential oils can be a great joy. The perception of the different fragrances, the mixing, the making, the playful approach to the substances can create a childlike delight in the preparer. Imagine the fine feeling of personally creating a wonderfully fragrant and effective cream, a mask, a body lotion, or a good perfume!

2 ❧ The Essential Oils

Essential Oils in Nature

Before turning to the "soul" of natural cosmetics—the essential oils themselves—let me offer here a general survey of these oils: where they are found in nature, how they are produced, and how they should be employed. Included here also is a discussion of the sense of smell, which plays such a key role in the use of fragrant essences in cosmetics.

Essential oils are highly volatile fragrant substances. The product of plant metabolism, they can be compared in function to blood in the human body. Their presence enables plants to exchange information with neighboring plants and other microorganisms; to attract insects (e.g., bees), and to defend themselves against animals and other plants. The common geranium, for example, is rarely attacked by insects because of the scent given off by its essential oil (even in the absence of blossoms). Certain plants can also prevent other plants from propagating in the near vicinity—a fact that the gardener can make use of to keep weeds out of the vegetable garden.

The essential oils are formed in the plant's cell nucleus and stored in the leaves, blossoms, berries, fruit skins, wood, bark, resin, and roots. More prescisely, the oil is found in the plant's oil cells (and ducts), resin cells (and ducts), oil glands, and gland hairs. For those readers who are not botanists or biologists, this system corresponds approximately to our system of arteries, veins, blood vessels, tissue, and cells, all of which contain blood, our human "essential oil." The essential oil moves throughout the plant in the course of the day, entering the roots, leaves, stem, or blossoms at various times according to what function these parts need to fulfill at that moment—much as blood will rush to a particular area of the body (e.g., to the stomach after food is taken in). This fact determines the best time to harvest any given plant. Since the oil will fundamentally be heavily concentrated in certain parts of the plant, only those segments are collected that contain particularly large amounts of oil. Hence the descriptions of specific oils in this book always indicate which parts of the plant are to be collected. For example, the essential oil of the jasmine plant is found in the blossoms at night. Thus jasmine blossoms are harvested during the early morning hours, before sunrise.

The Manufacturing Process

Of course you do not need to be aware of every detail of the manufacturing process in order to create your own natural cosmetics. But the study of what an "absolute oil" actually is and how it is obtained should be of interest if you work with essential oils either therapeutically or professionally.

The essential oil is well protected in the cells and ducts of the plant and needs to be drawn out. Any of various procedures can be used to break down the cell walls and extract the oil, depending on the structure of the plant material, the amount of oil contained in the plant, and the qualitative standards set for the end product.

Citrus oils are obtained through the inexpensive and gentle

procedure of *pressing*. They are not heated in the process and suffer no loss of quality or change in composition. Lemon, orange, bergamot, grapefruit, tangerine, and lime are obtained by pressing. (Lime can also be distilled.) The essences derived thereby are pure, free of residues, and inexpensive.

Plants that contain a very low proportion of essential oils or that contain delicate sensitive oils (which cannot be isolated safely through other procedures) or resinous, hardly volatile substances are obtained through *extraction*. This process involves the use of solvents such as hexane, petroleum ether, or toluene. Occasionally the extraction process is achieved under the use of gases such as butane or carbon dioxide. Blossoms (e.g., jasmine) are "softened" in the solvent and heated. From time to time the solvent is replaced. After the complete separation of the essential oils from the plant parts, the solvent and plant substances are removed by distillation, leaving a pastelike mass, known as "concrete," that contains the plant waxes, chlorophyll, and essential oils. Alcohol is then added to this mass and heated in order to separate the waxes. After cooling, the mixture is filtered, and through a further distillation the alcohol is removed. The clear, soluble (not completely residue-free) essential oil, also called "absolute oil" or "essence absolue," remains. (The extremely minimal residue is no cause for concern when extremely diluted amounts of essential oils are used in natural cosmetics.) Such oils are expensive, since the yield is minimal and the production costs are high.

Enfleurage is a less frequently used method for extracting fine blossom oils that are difficult to isolate. The freshly picked blossoms are spread out on glass plates that have been coated with animal fat. The fat absorbs the flower fragrance. The blossoms are constantly replaced until the fat cannot take on any more fragrance. Once it is totally saturated the fat is called *pomade*. The essential oil is then separated by adding alcohol, which ultimately evaporates, leaving an expensive essential oil, free from any residues.

The oldest and most gentle—and inexpensive—procedure for deriving pure, residue-free oil is *distillation*. A distinction is made between steam distillation and vacuum distillation (which involves the use of heat alone, without water). This procedure is used for plants with a large proportion of essential oils, such as peppermint, or when the goal is to derive an oil with as little damage to the oil as possible. Oils obtained in this manner are high in quality, pure, and less expensive than those derived through extraction.

Resins are obtained with solvents such as alcohol, toluene, or hydrochloric acid. The solvent and essential oil are separated through distillation, leaving behind a resinoid, an essential oil that still contains solvent residue. This residue is not a cause for concern when used in cosmetics, since it is a minimal amount and the essential oils are used in a highly diluted form.

Oils derived by extraction and enfleurage termed "absolute," "absolue," or "essence absolue" have a very strong fragrance. Among these are benzoin, cassia, oak moss, honey, hyacinth, jasmine, mimosa, narcissus, rose, tuberose, and violet.

Properties of Essential Oils

The consistency of essential oils ranges from watery (lavender oil, for example) to firm (from the rose "otto," for example). Their colors vary from mostly clear to dark brown, green, dark red, or blue. They dye fabrics readily, so it is best not to let clothing come in direct contact with them.

Although these substances or essences are called oils they are not fatty. They evaporate in the air with varying speeds and intensities and are highly sensitive to light (ultraviolet rays) and heat. For this reason such oils are best kept in dark brown bottles and stored in a cool place. Close the bottles tightly immediately after use, and never expose them to sunlight.

Bath, massage, and skin care oils containing essential oils should also be kept in dark brown bottles. It is not advisable to keep them in plastic bottles, which may cause chemical reactions with the natural substances. Store this pure, unadulterated gift of nature in natural containers of glass, porcelain, or clay. Should the essences come in contact with fire, they may ignite—a reaction that can easily be observed when a twist of orange peel is pressed over a candle or pine branches are tossed into the fireplace and the igniting oils crackle explosively.

Citrus oils can be stored for up to six months, after which they begin to deteriorate in effectiveness and intensity of scent. Other oils can be kept for years without any loss in effectiveness. Indeed, some fragrances mature in the bottle, like a good wine.

Essential oils are highly concentrated and cannot be compared with herbal extracts. That is why only extremely small amounts of essential oils are necessary for an optimal effect in your cosmetics. The yield of essential oils is generally low. To obtain 1/3 ounce— the amount commercially sold by most merchants to the consumer—requires as much as 6.6 pounds of marjoram, 8.8 pounds of clary sage, 22 pounds of rosemary, 1,100 pounds of rose petals, or 2,200 pounds of hyacinth blossoms!

Use in Natural Cosmetics

Essential oils must always be applied to the skin in diluted form, except when treating pimples, warts, athlete's foot, or wounds. (These exceptions are described in the specific recipes involved.) The oils should never be used near the eyes and are applied to the mucous membranes only in highly diluted form.

An important rule: Success in skin care or healing results not from using large amounts of oil or mixing many oils together, but rather from using small mixtures of the right oils.

A table of proportions is given on page 182. Please consider the amounts given in the following recipes as maximum figures; a useful rule of thumb is that it can never hurt to use less.

When choosing essential oils for your personal cosmetics, please read chapters 4 and 5 and review the tables on pages 82 and 157 to see which oils are the most suitable for your skin and hair type. Next, narrow down your choices to those oils whose fragrances you prefer. Finally, the oils can be combined according to degree of volatility and scent intensities (see pages 180–181): in this way the oils that evaporate more quickly can be "held back" with the slower oils so that the special scent of the composition is retained as long as possible. This is of particular interest when you create your own individual natural perfume.

Caution: Keep your essential oils out of the reach of children, since the ingestion of certain undiluted oils can lead to poisoning. Specific precautions that should be observed when using essential oils are listed below.

Skin irritations can occur when bath or body oils include any of the following ingredients:

basil	lemongrass
cajuput	melissa
camphor	orange
carnation	oregano
cedarwood	peppermint
cinnamon	pine
citronella	rosemary
clove	tea tree
eucalyptus	thyme
lemon	verbena

Sensitive skin is fundamentally irritated by these essences, but dosages higher than 4 drops in the bath or 5–10 drops in 2 oz. of vegetable oil can have an irritating effect on any skin type. (Other essential oils are also known to irritate the skin, but are not listed here since they are not used in cosmetics.) In cases of **high blood pressure**, hyssop, rosemary, sage, or thyme should only be used in small dosages as an ingredient in bath or body oils.

In cases of **epilepsy**, fennel, sage, thuja, or hyssop should only be used in small doses in the bath.

During **pregnancy** do not use the following oils in high doses in baths or body oils, since they have an abortive effect:

basil	juniper
camphor	myrrh
carrot seed	oregano
cedarwood	rosemary
clove	sage
frankincense	verbena
hyssop	

The following essential oils should only be used in low doses in the early months of pregnancy: clary sage, geranium, peppermint, rose, rosemary. Other oils, such as pennyroyal, sassafras, and clove, are also known to have an abortive effect but are not used in cosmetics. Finally, *toddlers* should only have minimal doses of essential oils in their baths and skin care oils.

Effects on Body and Psyche

Essential oils affect the body, mind, and psyche. Much as they work in plants, they stimulate human metabolism and transmit neurochemical "messages" to organs (skin), glands (hormones), or body systems (lymphatic, blood circulation, immune system). They maintain, heal, and regenerate the skin. They are antiseptic, fungicidal, bacteriostatic, and antibacterial, which means that they kill germs or prevent the further growth of bacteria and viruses. When used in cosmetics, essential oils have a direct effect on the skin, tissue, and fluid systems. Additionally, they stimulate the mind and emotions through the sense of smell. This special property of cosmetics based on essential oils explains their significance in holistic treatment.

A list of oils arranged according to their effects appears on pages 44–46. When considering ingredients for a mixture, consider these characteristics along with the oil's skin care and healing properties; bath and massage oils in particular can be created with their harmonizing effects in mind.

Essential oils penetrate the skin within 10 to 20 minutes, since they dissolve in the sebaceous matter. This is approximately the length of time needed with a mask, pack, compress, or aromatic bath. Through their fragrances, the oils directly affect the sense of smell. However, the sense of smell also protects us from constant stimulation, by telling the nerves to "switch off" if there is continual scent input. (This function does not apply to unpleasant smells, however.)

When the skin is rubbed or massaged, the essential oils affect the skin and tissue according to their permeability. The body's reaction to the neurochemical "messages" (triggered by essential oils as they enter the body through the skin and are absorbed by the blood) will depend upon the individual's metabolism and circulation. A person whose diet is vegetarian, rich in vitamins and minerals and well balanced, will clearly have a different metabolism and skin and hair structure from someone who rarely exercises and whose diet features fat, fast foods, alcohol, caffeine, and nicotine. Slow metabolism, poor digestion, sluggish and inadequate elimination, clogged and functionally inert skin—the symptoms of an unhealthy way of living and eating—prevent the quick penetration of the essential oils into the skin and the complete unfolding of their active ingredients. A body that is wholly occupied with eliminating toxins can only sustain its basic functions with great effort. It is hardly surprising that a subtle energy such as that provided by essential oils will have only a limited effect, or none at all, on that body.

In changing from synthetic commercial cosmetics to natural cosmetics, begin with cleansing the synthetic substances from your skin over a period of two weeks. Periodic masks and facial steam baths are the best means to do this. During this time the hair should also be thoroughly cleaned and treated with rinses and oil treatments. The effects of cosmetics with essential oils are dependent on the skin and hair's permeability, cleanliness, and receptivity to absorption—conditions that are promoted, again, by a healthy lifestyle and good nutrition. In many cases, an improvement of skin and hair condition can be noted after just one week.

Our Sense of Smell

The sense of smell plays a decisive role in the production and choice of natural cosmetics, since many scents have a clearly stimulating effect and can cause various psychological and physical reactions. Aromatherapy, an ancient natural healing method that has reemerged in recent years, deals specifically with the sense of smell and the effects of aromas on body and psyche. It uses the essential oils described in these pages, as well as many other oils.

The nose is the organ that tells you which oil has a pure fragrance, which scent you prefer in your cosmetics, or which perfume appeals to you. It is a completely normal reaction to want to open and sniff the jars, tubes, and bottles arrayed on cosmetic shelves, and a wise marketing staff will always provide "testers" to satisfy this desire. We can hardly imagine what these products would be like if a manufacturer of synthetic cosmetics added no fragrances or dyes, offering them instead as they had originally been produced! I suspect that sales would be rather low, even if such products were sold at a price reflecting their low production cost.

Fragrances are molecules that have separated from their carriers (plants, flowers, fruit, food, drink, people, objects, etc.) and float in the air. They reach our noses and are sucked in when we breathe. In the upper part of the nose, the molecules meet the olfactory mucous membrane with its receptors made of thousands of hairy sensory cells. These hairs, or cilia, function like nerve endings and register every scent on the basis of its specific chemical composition, electrical tension, and probably its infrared vibrations. The cilia can recognize and differentiate among thousands of smells, even among many different smells in turn, as well as among those that are extremely subtle, such as highly diluted fragrances in liquids. A trained nose can differentiate up to 10,000 scents!

The function of the sense of smell has not yet been completely explained. One theory says that there are five types of receptor cells (for flowery, camphoric, acrid, pungent, and putrid smells), which together function like a lock. When a molecule of smell approaches the lock, if the key (smell) fits, then the information about a certain scent is carried to the brain. But however the receptors identify the smell, the sensory stimulation is guided on through the olfactory bulb, an amplifier, and through the olfactory nerve to the limbic system in the brain.

The limbic system, the oldest part of our brain, was already present before the thinking brain developed. Within this system nerve impulses engage two important parts (amygdalae and hippocampus). These are the centers of memory, sexuality, sympathy, antipathy, creativity, and emotional reactions. Here the scent is compared to a known smell and given a label. At the same time, pictures and feelings from previous events, people, landscapes, and objects are associated with the scent information. We then in turn react emotionally and physically through our autonomous nervous system. In case you have not yet noticed: the body scent of a person close to you helps determine your feelings of liking or antipathy toward that person.

In the limbic system, the nerve impulse is led to the hypothalamus, which serves as the switching point for the transmittal of scent messages to other areas of the brain. The hypothalamus is also the control station for the pituitary gland (hypophysis). According to the scent data it receives, it conveys chemical messages to the blood stream. For example, the hypothalamus activates and releases hormones, regulates body functions, or signals the body that it needs more sexual hormones. Finally, the thalamus connects the scent information of the limbic system with the area of thinking and judgment. The whole process—from the perception of a smell by the olfactory mucous membrane to the corresponding gland secretion—takes place in a matter of split seconds.

Thus a simple inhalation of one or another scent can cause changes in the body, initiating any of various physiological processes according to the specific scent information received: the immune system is activated, the blood pressure changes, digestion is stimulated, saliva gathers in the mouth, and so on. This complex reaction of brain and body takes place whenever you groom yourself with aromatic cosmetics, take a fragrance bath, or use your natural perfume.

Fragrance information can cause us to become calm, lively, stimulated, euphoric, hungry, satiated, sleepy, active, or free of pain. Some examples: scents such as clary sage oil stimulate the thalamus in the brain to release encephalin, a neurochemical that creates a sense of euphoria and simultaneously gives pain relief. The fragrance of ylang-ylang stimulates the pituitary gland, which then releases a sexually stimulating neurochemical, endorphin. The scent of lavender, chamomile, or neroli stimulates the release of serotonin, which has a calming effect for fear, stress, aggravation, and sleeplessness.

The Essential Oils: A Descriptive List

The following thumbnail descriptions list skin care and healing characteristics, possibilities for use, fragrances, and other important properties of the oils that are called for in recipes throughout this book. The botanical names are important only in ordering the oils in a pharmacy or from a qualified merchant. Knowledge of their botanical names will allow you to ask for the exact type of oil desired since there are many different types of thyme, lavender, rose, and so on. Some merchants also stock oils under different names. Neroli, for example, is also called orange blossom. Note also that the information listed here on color and consistency may help in differentiating perfume oils or "stretched" oils from the pure, true oils.

Angelica Root
(Angelica archangelica)

Cultivated in Europe, the oil of angelica is derived from its dried or fresh roots, as the name implies. It is a thin, clear liquid. Angelica root is a highly effective healing oil, since it is antiseptic, antibacterial or bacteriostatic (prevents the further growth of bacteria), fungicidal, and suitable for treating infections, skin fungus, and healing wounds. It smells spicy, earthy, and musky.

Basil
(Ocinum basilicum)

This clear, thin liquid oil is derived through distillation from the blooming tips of the herb. It is cultivated in the United States, France, Italy, the Balkan countries, and Egypt. Basil is antiseptic and tones and clears the skin, increasing its resilience and sleekness. It can be used as a skin cleanser or toner in facial care, or added to oils and creams to the bath to stimulate the metabolism of greasy, tired, limp, and colorless skin. It has a slightly irritating effect and should therefore only be used in small amounts on sensitive skin. It causes a hot-cold feeling in baths. The fragrance of basil is penetratingly sweet, spicy, and similar to anise.

Benzoin/Styrax
(Styrax benzoin)

Benzoin is a resinoid derived through extraction from the resin of a tree native to Asia. The oil is clear and thin. It is antiseptic, deodorizing, soothing to irritated skin, and heals wounds, infections, and abscesses. It can be used for chapped skin, redness, and itching. In a diluted form, it can prevent the formation of blisters. A strong natural preservative, it can be used as such in all recipes (creams, ointments). Its scent, according to the country of its source, is balsamy, sweet, or warm.

Bergamot
(Citrus bergamia)

The greenish, thin oil of bergamot is obtained by pressing out the peel of a green bitter orange that grows in California, South America, Italy, Spain, and West Africa. An all-purpose oil for cosmetics, it can be used by every skin type and for many functional disturbances. It is antiseptic, slightly astringent, deodorizing, healing for wounds, and generally beneficial for the skin. It also helps in cases of dandruff, seborrhea, acne, herpes (lip blisters and genital herpes), shingles, eczema, excessive perspiration (armpits), and unpleasant body odor. Bergamot has a reducing effect on seborrhagia, greasy skin and hair, and oily seborrhea; the same is true for treating acne. Other areas of application are eczema, wound disinfection, and prevention of scar formation.

Bergamot goes with all bath oils, toners, deodorants, and perfumes. Its scent is fresh, sparkling, sweet, and clear. In case you are a tea drinker, you will recognize bergamot as the aroma of Earl Grey tea.

Bergamot tans the skin (like all citrus oils) and increases its sensitivity to light. For medium-strong UV rays, it should be applied with a vegetable oil 30 minutes before sunbathing. Where the UV rays are stronger, however, as they are in the mountains, at the seashore, or in the sun studio, caution is advised. One substance in the oil not only increases its sensitivity to light but is also phototoxic, which means it could in certain circumstances destroy cells due to strong UV influences. The result can be sunburn, redness, and spots that diminish only after several days.

Cajeput
(Melaleuca leucadendron)

This oil is derived through distillation from the fresh leaves and twig ends of a tree that grows in Australia, Indonesia, and Malaysia. Its oil, which smells like eucalyptus, is clear and thin.

Cajeput is antiseptic, antimicrobial, and eases pain. It is primarily applied in cases of skin pain, hair loss, and infection. Since it irritates sensitive skin, niaouli oil may be substituted instead.

Camphor
(Cinnamomum camphora)

Camphor oil is obtained through distillation of the wood of the camphor tree, which is found in Japan, China, India, Ceylon, and

Madagascar. It is thin and clear with a strong stimulating and healing effect on the skin.

Use this oil in small amounts only, since it is irritating to sensitive skin and has a slight reddening effect. However, it is quite suitable for oily skin, for general care and cleansing, and for the treatment of acne since it stimulates the metabolism and has a clearing effect. Blue spots or bruises, which women often develop even after minor contusions, can be treated very well with skin oil containing camphor. It also supports the healing of wounds, burns, and abscesses. The scent of camphor is medicinal and strong.

Carrot Seed
(Daucus carota)

The oil of the carrot seed primarily contains the well-known pigment carotene, but does not contain vitamins A, E, and provitamin A, which are found in the root. The thin, yellow oil is derived through distillation from ground seeds and is especially good for skin care.

Carrot seed oil stimulates cell renewal and also stimulates the sweat and sebaceous glands, which is of particular benefit to mature, dry skin and dry hair. Carrot seed is therefore an ideal oil for wrinkle creams and facial oils. It also protects and treats normal skin, as well as skin exposed to weather extremes. On the other hand, it should not be used for acne or oily skin. It offers limited protection against the sun in sun oils (together with sesame or hazelnut oil) and dyes the skin because of its carotene content. It can be mixed with almond oil to create an effective skin care oil. Its scent is woodsy, earthy, and fruity.

Cedarwood
(Cedrus atlantica, Juniperus virginiana, Juniperus mexicana)

Cedarwood oil is derived through distillation from the wood waste and sawdust of cedarwood. This tree can be found in the United States, North Africa, and the Near East. The oil is thin and clear.

Cedarwood is a general skin care oil that is antiseptic, astringent, soothing, and removes excess water. It is used in natural hair care products particularly for the treatment of greasy hair, dandruff and psoriasis, and for the treatment of acne, infections, rashes, eczema, dermatitis, and itching skin. It gently stimulates the skin. Because of its light wood, sweet-and-sour, and leather-like scent, it is often used in men's cosmetics and the corresponding perfumes. It is especially found in aftershave lotions because of its skin-soothing characteristics. It also serves as protection against insects.

Chamomile, Blue
(Matricaria chamomilla)

A plant native to Germany, blue chamomile is now cultivated also in Hungary, the Soviet Union, Egypt, and North America. It differs from the Roman chamomile in that it has a much higher proportion of azulene, which gives the essential oil a blue color. Azulene is very effective against infections and accelerates the healing process.

Only infections and wound inflammations should be treated with this relatively expensive oil. Otherwise, the blue chamomile has the same effects as Roman chamomile. However, its scent is stronger, almost intoxicatingly sweet, spicy-green, and slightly fruity.

Chamomile, Roman
(Anthemis nobilis)

Roman chamomile can be found in England, Bulgaria, Yugoslavia, France, and Hungary. A healing plant that has been known for thousands of years, its essential oil is distilled from the blossoms and the whole plant. The oil is yellowish, thin, and relatively expensive.

Its effect is antiseptic, vasoconstricting, healing and beneficial for skin and hair. Roman chamomile is used for sensitive, dry, reddened, or itchy skin, infected wounds, abscesses, acne, and rashes. It accelerates the healing of wounds and helps skin allergies when added to a cream or oil. Broken veins are said to be treated successfully with chamomile oil. It also makes raw, chapped hands smooth and supple. A chamomile rinse can be used to treat blond hair. Its relaxing fragrance is moderately sweet-sour and spicy-green.

Citronella
(Cymbopogon nardus)

This oil is derived from a reed-shaped grass that grows in China, Indonesia, and South America. It is mainly used in the manufacture of soaps, facial toners, and perfumes. Because of its cost, the cosmetic industry prefers to use melissa oil with its similar fragrance.

Citronella is fungicidal, antibacterial, and generally refreshing. It is an important component in all insect repellent preparations. It can be used for skin fungus and infections, as well as to add a refreshing aroma to bath water, perfumes, and homemade soaps. Some individuals may be allergic to citronella; for this reason, and because it is slightly irritating to the skin, use the oil in small amounts only. The scent is weakly sweet, forest-flowery, and rose-like (Java) or camphor-like (Ceylon).

Clary Sage
(Salvia sclarea)

This essential oil is derived through distillation from the blossoms of an herb that is cultivated in France, Spain, and the Soviet Union. It yields a thin light to yellowish liquid.

Clary sage has an estrogen-like and deodorizing effect. Its scent is euphoriant, relaxing, and aphrodisiac. It is similar to sage oil but has a milder effect. Clary sage is used for hydrated, infected, and normal skin, for hair care and dandruff, where it hastens the sloughing off of flakes by vitalizing the scalp. Its sweet smell is like hay and bergamot.

Clove Blossoms and Leaves
(Eugenia caryophyllata)

The clove tree grows in Indonesia, Tanzania, Madagascar, and Ceylon. Two types of clove oil with similar characteristics are obtained from its blossoms and leaves through distillation. The blossom oil is more expensive and has a warmer, spicier, and sweeter scent; by contrast, the leaf oil is not as fruity. Clove is very antiseptic and pain-relieving. Thus the thin, clear oil is used in many pain-relieving medications; its scent is familiar to everyone who has been to the dentist. Its use in natural cosmetics extends to warts, callouses, infected wounds, and insect stings. Since it is slightly caustic, it should always be used in small doses. One example of its use is in aftershave lotions, since its woody scent harmonizes well and it disinfects small razor-nicks.

Cypress
(Cupressus sempervirens)

This evergreen tree is an emblem of the Mediterranean region. A thin, clear oil is derived through distillation from its leaves, twigs, and cones. It smooths and tautens the skin, is astringent, deodorizing, vasoconstricting, and styptic. It reduces the amount of perspiration, which is why cypress oil can be used in a foot bath or special lotion to successfully treat sweaty feet. The oil is also suitable for the care of greasy, hydrated, slack, tired, and sluggish skin and for the treatment of varicose veins (see page 139). Cypress oil repels insects and has a fresh, lemony, and spicy scent—a pleasant fragrance for the bathtub. It is an important scent for men's cosmetics and perfumes.

Eucalyptus
(Eucalyptus globulus)

This thin clear to greenish-colored oil is obtained from the leaves and small twigs of the eucalyptus tree. It is characteristic for Australian flora, but also grows on the Iberian peninsula.

Eucalyptus oil is generally known for its strong antiseptic and healing effect on infections of the respiratory system. Since it easily irritates the skin, it is only used for inflammations, infectious wounds, and blisters (resulting from herpes, chicken pox, or drug allergy). Abscesses can also be treated with the oil. Finally, it can serve as an insect repellent. Eucalyptus has a slight estrogen-like effect on the body. Its fragrance is fresh and pungent.

Fennel
(Foeniculum vulgare)

Only the thin, yellowish oil of the sweet fennel seed is used in natural cosmetics and aromatherapy. It has a very mild effect. Fennel draws water from the body, stimulates the local circulation when used as an additive in body and massage oils, and contains estrogen-like phytohormones. It has a tautening effect on the skin, strengthens the muscle tone, and increases the elasticity of the connective tissue and the skin. Fennel is therefore used to treat mature skin, wrinkles, furrows, weakness of the connective tissue and cellulite, and to maintain the gums. An ingredient in many products for oral and dental care, it has a pleasant taste in homemade toothpaste and helps to heal infections in the area of the mouth. The scent of the essential oil is like that of the kitchen herb or the tea.

Frankincense
(Boswellia carterii)

The oil of the boswellia tree, which grows wild in Arabia, is distilled from the resin. Frankincense has been used for thousands of years by the Arabian people. It was already used in Egypt during the time of the pharaohs for skin care and the preservation of the corpses of rulers.

The thin, clear-to-yellowish oil is astringent, rejuvenating, and extremely beneficial to the skin. It is not only used specifically for mature skin and wrinkles, but also for raw, chapped skin, hand care, and the healing of wounds. Typical of the warm, balsamy oil is its fragrance of lemon and conifer. It is suitable for creating perfumes with a woody, tart character, and equally appropriate for fresh, lemon-like mixtures. It blends well with myrrh to create a facial oil for mature skin. Frankincense also harmonizes well with wood fragrances. The oil sold under the name of "olibanum" is identical to frankincense oil.

Garlic
(Allium sativum)

The thick, light oil of the garlic root is obtained through distillation and has its own characteristic penetrating scent. Of course, garlic is not used in the preparation of creams, but the substances it contains make it an indispensable healing oil for the treatment of warts, calluses, abscesses, scabs, and corns (in which case it is always used undiluted), as well as noninflamed abscesses and infected wounds. It is strongly antiseptic, fungicidal, detoxifying, and healing for wounds.

Geranium
(Perlargonium graveolens)

The same common geranium that blooms so splendidly in gardens and flowerpots contains a valuable essential oil for skin care, a clear, thin liquid that is obtained from the leaves and stem through distillation. Geranium oil is antiseptic, astringent, deodorizing, toning, anti-inflammatory, cleansing, and stimulates the lymphatic system. It can occasionally provoke an allergic reaction. Such sensitization is rare, however; indeed, the essential oil of the geranium is recommended for general skin care—for dry as well as oily skin—since the oil has a balancing effect on sebaceous production. Geranium oil is very much to be recommended for sluggish, oily skin.

Further areas of use are: weakness of the connective tissue, cellulite, seborrhea, acne, abscesses, bleeding, infections, dry eczema, herpes, and shingles. Geranium oil is said to stimulate breast growth when mixed with ylang-ylang in a body oil and used regularly. It is also an insect repellent. The fragrance is rosy-minty and harmonizes well with rose and rosewood.

Hyssop
(Hyssopus officinalis)

Hyssop is an antiseptic oil for healing obtained from the stems and blossoms of an herb that grows wild in the Mediterranean region. It can be used to treat eczema and other skin conditins, infections, bruises (as a warm compress), and shock injuries (as a cold compress). Its scent is sweet, spicy, woody, and camphor-like.

Immortelle
(Helichrysium angustifolium DC)

This wild-growing evergreen herb, also known as the Italian
strawflower, can be found throughout the Mediterranean region.
The oil, derived from the blossoms, is thin and clear. It is anti-
inflammatory, fungicidal, and astringent. It soothes burns and
smoothes raw, chapped skin. Immortelle is used as a fixative in
perfumes. Its fragrance is intense, honey-like, sweet, and fruity with
a light touch of chamomile.

Jasmine
(Jasminum grandiflorum, J. officinale)

Jasmine oil has been used for thousands of years in skin care
cosmetics and perfumes. The bush originally grew in East India,
but can also be found today also in southern France, Spain, Morocco, Algeria, and Egypt. The reddish-brown oil is derived from
the blossoms through extraction and is very expensive. Often it can
be obtained more economically when it is diluted with a vegetable
oil (10% solution), whereby its intensity of scent is decreased and
its effectiveness reduced. This stretched oil may be acceptable for
the production of perfume, but pure jasmine oil is absolutely
necessary for cosmetics. Despite its price, do not shy away from
jasmine: only very small—and thus affordable—amounts are ever
needed for homemade cosmetics.

Jasmine oil is good for the care for all types of skin. It is toning
and antiseptic, and has a relaxing, aphrodisiac scent. It is particularly
suited for treating dry, sensitive, and sore skin. It has a soothing
effect on skin infections; like all blossom oils, it has a strong affinity
for facial skin. A bath with jasmine oil lets you forget aggravation,
stress, anger, nervousness, and worries. Jasmine oil lends many
perfumes a flowery, honey-sweet, fruity touch.

Juniper
(Juniperus communis)

The berries of the juniper bush which grows throughout Europe are distilled to obtain the thin, clear liquid called juniper oil or juniper berry oil.

Juniper purifies the blood, promotes metabolism, is antiseptic, detoxifying, toning, astringent, and anti bacterial. It tightens tissue and inhibits infections. It is particularly suited for cleansing the skin in the form of aromatic lotions or cleansing oil, and for the care of oily, hydrated, or sluggish skin. The skin will be taut and well supplied with blood after a juniper-oil facial cleanser or facial steam bath.

Further areas of use are: dental care, cleansing of wounds, and treatment of acne, psoriasis, dermatitis, and infections. Juniper oil draws out fluids and therefore also appears in cellulite recipes. Its scent is powerful, and slightly reminiscent of pine needles—the typical gin scent.

Lavender
(Lavendula officinalis, L. vera)

There are many different kinds of lavender, each with its own chemical composition and scent; the fragrance of English lavender, for example, is different from that of lavender indigenous to southern France. In choosing "your" lavender, let your nose be the guide. Lavender grows throughout the Mediterranean region as well as in England, the Soviet Union, and Australia. The fresh stems and flower buds are used to make the essential oil.

Lavender is an all-purpose oil for skin care. Its effect is antibacterial, pain-relieving, healing for wounds, soothing for skin diseases, deodorizing, antiseptic, fungicidal, insect-repellent, rejuvenating, and anti-inflammatory. It may be used to treat all types of skin and is effective for acne and oily hair (as it regularizes sebum production), itchy skin, hand care, cracked skin, bruises, shock injuries (in ice-cold compresses), acne scars, blisters, abscesses, furuncles, warts, boils, eczema, athlete's foot (tea tree is more effective here, however), wounds, and burns. A bath with lavender soothes and heals the skin after a sunburn.

Since it has proven itself to be one of the most effective oils in natural cosmetics, you will find lavender in almost all the recipes in the following chapter. It also plays an important role in aromatherapy, for its fragrance has a calming and relaxing effect. Headaches disappear with cold lavender compresses. In addition, lavender strengthens the effects of other oils in the mixture, which is why it is never wrong to add some lavender. Its scent is sweet, balsamy, flowery, woodsy, and light.

Lemon
(Citrus limonum)

Lemon oil is obtained by cold pressing pure, untreated lemon peels. It is a thin liquid with a clear color. This essential oil is astringent, antibacterial, and antiseptic; it cleanses and cares for the skin and rejuvenates the cell.

Since it contains citronellol, lemon has a slightly irritating effect, particularly on sensitive skin. It is used for oily, sluggish skin and the treatment of acne. The oil reduces sebaceous production, and clears and tautens the skin. This last effect is also beneficial for tired and aging skin. An ashen face is easily freshened by lemon, since it stimulates the skin functions. Lemon bleaches well and can therefore be used to treat freckles (but only in diluted form). It has also proven itself effective in treating brittle fingernails and for general hand care.

Further areas of use are: blond hair care, itching, herpes, scabs, wounds (lemon stimulates the formation of white blood cells), warts, furuncles, frostbite, insect stings, nosebleeds, and bleeding gums. Lemon increases the light sensitivity of the skin and is therefore used in tanning agents (see the section on bergamot, page 24). The oil has the typical fresh, sparkling scent of lemon.

Lemongrass
(Cymbopogon flexousus, C. citratus)

This oil is mentioned because of its refreshing fragrance and deodorizing qualities, which are repellent to insects. It is derived from a grass native to India, China, and South America.

It can be used to prepare an invigorating summer bath, to repel insects, to give perfume a fresh lemon-verbena touch, and to bathe sweating feet. The oil irritates sensitive skin and should be used only in small doses in preparations for this skin type.

Melissa (Lemon Balm)
(Melissa officinalis)

This plant is a well-known ingredient in herbal remedies and folk medicine. Its clear, thin oil is relatively expensive, since the yield from the distillation of the plant is not very high. The oil contains citronellol, which can cause slight skin irritation. Melissa should therefore only be used in 1% dilutions. Yet it is definitely suitable for general skin and hand care and for skin allergies, and has proven to be very effective in the treatment of herpes blisters when applied to the blisters in undiluted form. Melissa oil stimulates the metabolism and tones and enlivens the skin through its mildly irritating effect. In aromatic baths and creams it has a cooling effect; it can also be used in small amounts to treat sunburn. It is also used in natural insect repellant formulas. The scent is strong, herbal-sweet, and lemony.

Myrrh
(Commiphora molmol abyssinica)

Myrrh is a desert tree that grows in North Africa, Somalia, and Ethiopia. The thick, reddish-brown oil is obtained through extraction and distillation of its resin. Myrrh has a powerful healing effect on wounds, as if it contained the strength and energy of the intense African sun. The ancient Egyptians used it in their ointments and creams and as an embalming agent to preserve the corpses of the pharaohs. It is easy to understand why we still use it today for the care of mature skin.

Myrrh oil is rejuvenating, fungicidal, anti-inflammatory, antiseptic, cooling, and astringent. As a major component in ointment or cream, it can be used to treat skin that is rough, cracked, chapped, or infected, including facial skin, and is recommended for scabs, oozing eczema, abscesses (even ulcers in the mouth), skin fungus, and athlete's foot. It can also be added to mouthwash to treat bad breath, gum problems, and fistula in the mouth. Its scent is warm, spicy, balsamy, and sweet—a pleasant oriental fragrance that may be included in strong perfume mixtures.

Myrtle
(*Myrtus communis*)

Myrtle oil is distilled from the blossoms and twig tips of a tree native to the Mediterranean region. It is a thin, clear liquid with a fresh and slightly herbal fragrance. Myrtle is astringent, antiseptic, and antibacterial; it may be used for general skin care and acne.

Neroli or Orange Blossom
(*Citrus aurantium*)

One of the loveliest blossom oils, neroli is obtained from the flowers of the bitter orange tree as they open. This tree is also the source of petitgrain oil (see page 39). It grows in southern France, Morocco, Algeria, and Egypt. The oil got its name from an Italian princess who used it as her favorite perfume. The thick, brownish oil has a spicy, sweet-bitter scent. The fragrance is extremely intense and lasts for a long time. This oil can be used in very small amounts in perfume with no diminution of its effect.

Neroli rejuvenates, smoothes and treats the skin, relieves skin pain, and is nonirritating. It is especially suitable for dry and mature skin. Since the oil stimulates cell renewal, it can be added to healing oils for treating wounds (e.g., acne lesions) and to promote healing of deep cuts that have closed. Its scent is calming and at the same time has a certain aphrodisiac quality that provides an interesting note in bath oils or perfumes. This oil is not cheap, but is well worth including in any collection of essential oils.

Orange blossom water is closely related to neroli, since it is obtained from the blossoms of the same tree. The aromatic water is astringent and, added to face lotion or a cream, is good for dry, sensitive skin. The water and the oil can naturally be combined to provide a wonderfully harmonic scent in natural cosmetics.

Niaouli
(Melaleuca viridifolia)

Niaouli (niauli) is derived through distillation from the leaves and twig tips of a tree native to Asia and Australia.

It is strongly antiseptic and antibacterial, and so can be used to treat acne, infections, minor injuries, and light burns. It clears and cleanses the skin, stimulating rejuvenation. Its scent is eucalyptus-like, fresh, and spicy.

Onion
(Allium cepa)

The light essential oil derived from the well-known onion serves the purpose of healing. Theoretically it could also be used to treat the skin—but who would want to make a body oil or facial cream permeated by its typical, intensive onion smell?

However, onion oil is strongly antiseptic and anti-bacterial and inhibits inflammation. It can be used it on skin infections, abscesses, warts, frostbite, ulcers, burns, and to care for chapped skin. It bleaches the skin and can be used in a diluted form to treat freckles.

Orange (Sweet)
(Citrus aurantium)

Natural cosmetic products use the sweet orange oil of trees cultivated in the United States, the Mediterranean region, South Africa, and Brazil. (Note that this oil is to be distinguished from the oil of the bitter orange tree, which gives us neroli and petitgrain.) Sweet orange oil is derived from the fresh, untreated fruit peels through cold pressing.

Orange is slightly astringent and used for general skin care (particularly for oily skin in the case of acne), cellulite, and bad breath because of its pleasant taste and smell. A few drops of orange in a facial lotion has a very refreshing and stimulating effect on the skin.

Orange oil is also ideal for a child's bath or baby oil. It increases the light sensitivity of the skin to ultraviolet rays (see under berga-mot, page 24). It has a very refreshing, sweet, slightly tart scent that makes a summer bath even more enjoyable, particularly when mixed with lemon and bergamot. However, orange should be used in small doses only, since it does irritate the skin.

Parsley
(Petroselinum sativum, P. hortense)

This thick, light to greenish-yellow oil is obtained through distillation of the entire plant and seeds of this kitchen herb.

Its effect is cleansing, toning, slightly stimulating, and vasoconstricting. This last characteristic is useful in the treatment of the skin marred by the fine red veins that are a result of broken capillaries. The oil prevents the expansion of the veins and may even shrink them so much over a long course of treatment that they are no longer visible. It is also used in natural cosmetic products for oily, impure, and tired skin, as well as for cellulite. Its fragrance is the typical spicy scent of the kitchen herb.

Patchouli
(Pogostemon cablin)

This aphrodisiac oil is derived through distillation of the dried and fermented leaves of a bush that grows in Indonesia, China, and Madagascar. It is dark yellow to brown in color and thick in consistency. Patchouli contains patchoulene, a substance that, like the azulene found in blue chamomile, is a healing agent for inflamed skin and wounds.

Patchouli oil is anti-inflammatory, toning, antiseptic, fungicidal, and stimulates cell regeneration. It is recommended for use in caring for mature skin; acne; skin which is hydrated, raw, chapped, and scaly; dandruff; and in treating wounds, fungus infections, and eczema. Patchouli has a heavy, balsamy-sweet, woody, earthy scent. It is a good basic component in strong perfume, and clings to the clothes for weeks.

Peppermint
(Mentha piperita)

This familiar herb grows worldwide today. Its thin, clear oil is derived from the herb through distillation. It contains menthol, a crystalline substance that is known for its ability to open the breathing passages.

In cosmetics, peppermint oil is used for cleansing, since it is slightly antiseptic, anti-inflammatory, and toning. It purifies sluggish skin and pores and can activate the skin when used in a facial steam bath. Peppermint oil is entirely suitable for the treatment of oily skin, acne and blackheads; it can also be applied undiluted to pimples. Further areas of use are for itchy skin, infections, and dandruff. It has a generally refreshing and stimulating effect on the scalp when added to shampoo.

Because peppermint oil is slightly irritating to the skin, caution in its use is advisable. Use at most three or four drops in an aromatic bath, and add it only sparingly to body and facial oils. It creates a hot-cold effect in the bath, making the hot water feel cold—a pleasant effect when the skin is sunburned. Try a mixture of 6 parts lavender to 4 parts peppermint for a healing bath. To check for sensitivity, test the oil on the underside of the arm, where the skin is usually as sensitive as that of the face. The fragrance of peppermint is typically fresh.

Petitgrain
(Citrus aurantium)

This oil is derived from the leaves of the bitter orange tree (see under neroli page 36) through distillation. Its chemical composition and scent are similar to that of neroli, but have a lighter touch.

Although it is slightly deodorizing, petitgrain is primarily used in cosmetics for its refreshing, flowery-sweet scent. Examples of its use are in hair tonics (in combination with rosemary), aromatic baths, body oils, and in perfumes. Petitgrain costs less than neroli, but does not have the strong rejuvenating effect of the latter; thus it should be chosen over neroli only where its lighter fragrance is specifically preferred.

Pine Needle
(Abies sibirica ledeb)

This thin, clear oil is derived through steam distillation from the needled branches of the pine tree. It is excellent not only for use as a sauna oil but also for the treatment of intense sweating of the feet, since it has strong antiseptic and deodorizing qualities.

I know no direct skin care benefits of this oil, but I recommend its use as a bath oil in cases of nervousness, stress, or mental exhaustion—states that can have a harmful effect on the skin with time. Pine oil is slightly irritating to the skin and has the typical spicy pine fragrance.

Rose
(Rosa damscena, R. otto, R. gallica, R. centifolia, R. alba)

The "queen" of flowers, the rose is also the queen or mother of fragrances. The oil of the rose has been valued as a cosmetic, healing substance, and perfume for thousands of years by all of the peoples of the Old World, the Far East, and India. This aphrodisiac oil is obtained through extraction from the various types of rose petals mentioned above. It is a thick reddish-brown to greenish-orange liquid. When it is derived from the "otto" rose, its consistency is pasty to solid at room temperature. The steam distillation process is also used for the Bulgarian damascena rose. After distillation, the solution that remains is pure rose water.

Rose oil is astringent, toning, antiseptic, styptic, anti-inflammatory, and rejuvenating. It is particularly good for dry, sensitive, and mature skin, yet it can be used in almost every recipe for all skin types. Treatment with diluted rose oil over a longer period of time can help in the case of ruptured blood vessels and broken capillaries. Its multiple effects make it a highly valuable ingredient in natural skin care products, well worth its imposing cost. Finally, rose fragrance will provide the "basis" of all rosy, flowery, and aphrodisiac scents in natural perfumes.

An economical replacement for rose oil is rose water, a solution derived from the rose blossoms during the oil's manufacturing process. Its effect is also toning, antiseptic, astringent, and calming for inflamed skin. It can be added to virtually any recipe and is also recommended as a pure facial lotion for all skin types.

Rosemary
(Rosmarinus officinalis)

The essential oil of this kitchen herb is derived from the entire blossoming herb through distillation. It is thin and clear. The cosmetic and medicinal use of rosemary goes back to the time of the ancient Greeks.

Rosemary is beneficial in the loss or thinning of hair, loss or change of hair color (but don't expect any dramatic changes with rosemary), dandruff, and cellulite. The astringent and antiseptic properties of rosemary oil stimulate tissue circulation, the metabolism of the skin, and lymph drainage. The oil is highly effective in facial lotions, cleansing creams, body toners, shampoos, hair rinses, and aromatic baths. A rosemary bath is stimulating and warming, whether in the form of a wake-up morning bath or a refreshing bath at the start of a long evening. Its fragrance is woodsy, herb-like, and similar to lavender. It is often a surprise for the inexperienced nose to encounter the difference in fragrance between the herb and the oil.

Rosewood
(Aniba rosaedora)

This oil is derived through distillation from the wood of a Brazilian tree that is not related in any way to the rose flower. Yet its scent is slightly rosy, flowery, and spicy-sweet, so that the less expensive rosewood oil can be used in perfume mixtures, lotions, or soaps as a replacement for rose oil.

Rosewood oil is antibacterial, slightly toning, and mild in effect. It makes the skin smooth and supple, and is suitable for every skin type. Used in body oils, it has a deodorizing effect. Even weakness of the connective tissue has been successfully treated with rosewood oil. It is also used to treat dark hair.

Sage
(Salvia officinalis)

Sage oil is derived from the entire plant; it is indigenous to the southern European countries, particularly Yugoslavia and Greece. It was already known as a folk medicine to the Greeks and Romans, who gave it the name *herba sacra* ("holy herb"). Another form of sage oil, different in chemical composition, is obtained from *Salvia lavandulae folia*, which grows wild throughout the entire Mediterranean region. In fact, some 450 different types of sage are known on the earth; my discussion here pertains only to the Dalmantinian sage oil, however.

Sage is antiseptic, reduces excessive perspiration, and stimulates the circulation. It contains an estrogen-like active ingredient with a tautening effect, making this oil ideal for aging skin. Because of its strength, it should be used sparingly and selectively. In shampoos and hair oils, sage serves to eliminate functional disturbances. It has also proved itself effective against infections and for healing wounds. Its scent is strong, spicy, reminiscent of herbs and camphor. To prevent any possibility of skin irritation and to avoid the slightly toxic effect of the thujone contained in sage oil, try substituting the milder clary sage (see page 28).

Sandalwood
(Santalum album, S. citrinum, S. spicatum)

The oil of the sandalwood tree of Southeast Asia has long been known as both perfume and medicinal agent. This thick, brownish to yellow liquid is antiseptic, slightly astringent, soothing, somewhat rejuvenating, and aphrodisiac. It can be used to care for all types of skin, especially raw, infected, oily, or dry skin (warm compresses are particularly good here); it has also proved itself in the treatment of itchy skin and acne. Added to hair oils, shampoos, and rinses, it grooms dark hair and imparts a silky shine.

Sandalwood's sweet, warm, woody-balsamy scent can be found in many classic oriental and aphrodisiac perfumes (such as "Shalimar").

It is well suited to men's cosmetics such as aftershave lotions, creams, or facial lotions. I prefer it as a base for my facial oil.

Tea Tree
(Melaleuca alternifolia)

This healing oil is derived though distillation from the leaves and young twigs of a tree that is primarily native to Australia. Its chemical composition is similar to that of eucalyptus and rosemary oil. The subject of much research, the thin yellowish oil is now known throughout the world for its highly disinfectant, fungicidal, bactericidal, and virucidal properties. It is effective against all kinds of fungus infections; all infections including candida; herpes blisters; warts; abscesses; acne (as a skin cleanser and acne cream with jojoba), and pimples (apply undiluted). To prevent athlete's foot after swimming at a public pool, apply a tea tree foot oil or tea tree in a water solution.

The tea tree oil is also used in shampoos and rinses. It stimulates the functions of the scalp and has a cleansing, clearing effect. The oil should be used sparingly in healing baths since it can irritate sensitive skin. It is absolutely nontoxic. The tea tree scent is fresh and reminiscent of camphor.

Thyme
(Thymus vulgaris)

The clear, thin essential oil of the thyme plant, known throughout the Mediterranean region as a folk medicine for millennia, is derived from the entire blossoming herb through distillation. Many varieties of the plant are known.

Thyme oil is strongly antiseptic and antibacterial, supports the circulatory system and metabolism, raises blood pressure, and inhibits infections. It is used in natural cosmetics for the treatment of sluggish, oily skin, and is a natural healing agent for wounds and infections, since it stimulates the formation of white blood cells. Thyme oil can be used in gargle solutions and mouthwashes and can be added to toothpaste to care for the teeth and gums. Its activating effect on the scalp is useful in shampoos, hair oils, treatments, rinses, and lotions to prevent hair loss. Its stabilizing effect on the adrenal cortex also indirectly influences the skin. (Functional disturbances of the adrenal cortex affect estrogen activity, which is responsible for skin and muscle tone.) The fragrance of thyme is herb-like and sweet.

Ylang-ylang
(Canaga odorata)

This precious oil is derived through distillation of the blossoms of a tree native to the Comoro Islands and Madagascar. It is a medium thick, yellowish-green oil with an intense scent.

In natural cosmetics ylang-ylang is used to care for both dry and oily skin, since it has a balancing effect on sebaceous production. A toning blossom oil, it is suitable for all skin types. The fragrance is aphrodisiac, jasmine-like, heavy, sweet, and extremely intense, so that it can be used only in small doses in cosmetics and aromatic baths. Ylang-ylang gives many fragrance compositions a flowery warmth.

The following table provides a summary of the essential oils.

Effects of Essential Oils	astringent	antibacterial	antiseptic	aphrodisiac	bacteriostatic	deodorant	disinfectant	healing for skin	hormone-like	insect repellent	irritating	protective	reddening	rejuvenating	relaxing	stimulating	tanning	toning	water removing	wound healing
Angelica Root	•	•		•																
Anise											•									
Basil																•				
Benzoin						•	•													
Bergamot		•				•	•								•			•		•
Cajeput										•										

Effects of Essential Oils	astringent	antibacterial	antiseptic	aphrodisiac	bacteriostatic	deodorant	disinfectant	healing for skin	hormone-like	insect repellent	irritating	protective	reddening	rejuvenating	relaxing	stimulating	tanning	toning	water removing	wound healing
Calendula																				•
Camphor												•	•			•			•	•
Cardamom				•								•				•				
Carrot Seed												•								
Cedarwood	•							•		•						•				
Chamomile, Blue								•								•				•
Chamomile, Roman								•								•				•
Cinnamon	•	•	•	•	•		•													
Citronella										•										
Clary Sage				•		•		•	•							•				
Clove		•	•		•		•			•						•				
Coriander																•				
Cypress	•				•														•	
Eucalyptus		•	•		•	•	•	•	•	•	•					•				
Fennel									•										•	
Frankincense	•														•					
Garlic		•	•		•															
Geranium	•							•		•									•	•
Ginger																•				
Ginseng				•																
Hyssop		•	•		•															
Grapefruit						•														
Immortelle	•							•												
Jasmine				•				•							•			•		
Juniper	•	•	•	•	•		•	•						•		•		•	•	•
Lavender		•	•		•	•	•	•		•					•	•				•
Lemon	•	•	•		•							•			•		•	•		
Lemongrass									•			•								

Effects of Essential Oils	astringent	antibacterial	antiseptic	aphrodisiac	bacteriostatic	deodorant	disinfectant	healing for skin	hormone-like	insect repellent	irritating	protective	reddening	rejuvenating	relaxing	stimulating	tanning	toning	water removing	wound healing
Limette																		•		
Marjoram															•					
Melissa										•					•					
Myrrh	•							•						•	•					•
Myrtle	•	•	•		•															
Neroli				•	•										•					
Niaouli		•	•		•		•	•												
Nutmeg											•									
Onion		•	•	•	•															
Orange	•														•		•			
Parsely	•	•	•													•		•		
Patchouli				•			•							•	•			•		
Pennyroyal										•										
Pepper				•								•				•				
Peppermint							•	•	•							•		•		
Petitgrain						•														
Pine Needle		•	•	•	•	•														
Rose	•							•						•	•					
Rosemary	•															•				•
Rosewood		•	•		•										•					
Sage	•					•			•							•				•
Sandalwood	•			•				•						•	•					
Sassafras										•							•			
Savory		•	•		•															
Tea Tree		•	•		•	•					•									
Thyme		•	•		•	•					•					•				•
Tuberose				•																
Vanilla				•											•					
Verbena												•					•			
Ylang-ylang				•											•					

Quality and Cost

The quality of the essential oils used in any preparation is an important consideration, since only the pure, natural oils can actually elicit the desired effects in the human body. Unfortunately, even health food and natural cosmetic stores may offer oil products that have been stretched with some vegetable oil such as olive oil, synthesized chemically (so that they are not even partially derived from the plant they are named for), or created from a mixture of essences with a similar scent. Similarly adulterated perfume oils are also widely available. This deplorable state is supported by a cycle of profit greed on the part of manufacturers and an uncritical attitude on the part of consumers.

Synthetic oils are, of course, mainly manufactured in order to allow the industry to mass-produce perfumes and cosmetics inexpensively. Synthetic fragrances are also used in the manufacture of foods, consumer goods, detergents, and cleaning agents. (To be sure, if natural essences were used in all these products, virtually no affordable essential oils would be left over for cosmetic production.)

Still, the synthetic oils have no vital power and simply cannot be used to make natural cosmetics. Nor, in my experience, do they have the same effect on the sense of smell as pure oils. The stretched or mixed oils do retain a certain vital power, but these adulterated substances are unpredictable in effect.

To test oil for purity, try the following:
1. Rub a few drops of oil between two fingers. If it feels oily or greasy, it has probably been stretched with olive oil or almond oil.
2. Put a drop of oil on a piece of paper. If a greasy spot remains after evaporation, the oil has been stretched.
3. Put a drop of the essential oil in a glass of water. If the oil breaks up and even leaves a milky trace, it is probably a synthetic oil to which emulsifiers have been added. (Emulsifiers make the essential oil and vegetable oil water-soluble.)

4. If the oil smells like alcohol (i.e., like hard liquor), it has
   been stretched with ethyl alcohol. With some practice, your
   nose will soon be able to discriminate between pure and
   adulterated or stretched oils.

There is a further—and perhaps most simple—way to discriminate between oils bearing the same name, for here the product's
quality will naturally be reflected in its price. A pure, natural oil
made from organically grown plants will always be more expensive
than its synthetic or stretched counterpart.

3 Basic Ingredients for Natural Cosmetics

The Basic Ingredients: A List

Having surveyed the essential oils, here is a look at the carrier substances of skin and hair care oils necessary to make creams, lotions, toners, soaps, shampoos, and so on.

Agar-agar

This substance is made from seaweed and can be purchased as a powder or in stick form (mostly in health food stores). Like gelatin, agar-agar thickens liquids and thus can be used in recipes for products such as shampoos and shower gels.

Almond Bran

The dry residue of sweet almonds, a by-product made in the

process of obtaining almond oil, is used in rubbing masks (or "facial scrubs"), which remove the upper, dead skin layer. Make a paste of almond bran and water, then gently rub the facial skin with it.

Aloe Vera

Aloe vera has been used for thousands of years as a medicinal plant. The oldest reference to it is found on a papyrus roll from 1500 B.C. Javanese women rub aloe vera into their scalps in order to stimulate hair growth. In Greece (fourth century B.C.) the wounds of Alexander the Great were treated with this plant.

Aloe vera contains a gel that liquifies when it comes in contact with air. The plant's leaves are so well protected by their waxy coating against the loss of fluids that the plants can live for months in the desert without moisture. For injuries, burns, and skin problems, pluck a leaf from the plant and spread the exuding liquid on the afflicted area. The juice or gel contains important healing substances for the skin—steroids, organic acids (amino acids), enzymes, and polysaccharides. The regenerative qualities of aloe vera thus make it suitable for the treatment of the skin and hair and effective against acne. Premature aging of the skin, wounds, burns, gum diseases, and seborrhea can also be treated with aloe vera, as can hair loss resulting from seborrhea, dandruff, and damage to the nervous system.

Aloe vera should always be used fresh and pure—fresh because the product loses its effectiveness after six weeks; pure, because the addition of chemical preservatives, dyes, chemical emulsifying agents, and the like destroy the effectiveness of the natural substances. You can use liquid or gel-like aloe vera in hand-washing gels, healing ointments, packs, masks, moisturizing creams or lotions, shampoos, hair conditioners, and rinses. Aloe vera is also added to sun protection creams.

Alum

Made from lava stone, alum is slightly disinfecting, strongly astringent, and dissolves in warm water. It is used in cosmetics because of its astringent character.

Arnica Oil
(Arnica montana)

Arnica oil or tincture, derived through distillation from a flower native to Europe, is light to yellowish in color; its scent is spicy, woodsy, and earthy. Arnica tincture contains the vitamins A, B, C, and D.

This invigorating oil is an excellent healing agent for wounds. Arnica is a component in massage oils used for cellulite, since it activates the metabolism of the skin and tissue. Muscle strains and sprains can be treated with arnica compresses, and shock injuries and bruises with arnica ointment or oil. Arnica accelerates the dissolution of hematoma in tissue.

Arnica is also good for treating the skin and recommended when it is chapped, cracked, or scaly. Wounds that are healing poorly and abscesses can also be treated with arnica. The amount of oil should be limited to a 0.5% solution.

Avocado Oil

Avocado oil is derived from the flesh of a fruit that grows in tropical and subtropical zones, particularly Central America and California. Since it is similar to sebaceous fat, the oil quickly merges with it. About 20,000 IU of vitamin A, 40,000 IU of vitamin C, 300 IU of vitamin E, 2% protein, 8% carbohydrates, and amino acids, chlorophyll, linolenic acid, and histidine are contained in 2.2 pounds of avocado oil. Its healing qualities regenerate skin that has been damaged by parasites, soothes eczema, and promotes the regeneration of scarred skin. It treats scaly and dry skin and scalp, stimulates the growth of hair, and makes hard tissue soft and smooth. Avocado oil is used in massage and body oils because of its effect on body tissue and is added to facial and hair oils because of its benefits for the skin. The unsaturated fatty acids of the avocado make it useful as a light ultraviolet filter in sun protection oils as well. The pureed fruit is a valuable addition to masks and packs. If at all possible, use only cold-pressed oils.

Beeswax

Beeswax derived from honeycomb is naturally yellow in color; white beeswax, which has been bleached by air and sun, can cause allergies. Beeswax is a natural emulsifying agent that can make creams and lotions either smooth or hard, according to the proportion used. Together with borax, it can bind and stabilize emulsions that contain a great amount of oil. The yellow wax tints creams a golden yellow.

Bolus Alba

This white, powdery clay substance can be used to prepare facial masks. It detoxifies and tautens the skin, and thus is an effective remedy for impure skin and acne.

Borax

Borax is a white, natural mineral powder that makes water softer and gentler to the skin. Add a little pinch to water for sensitive, fatty, or impure skin or oily hair. It can also be added to cosmetics such as body lotions. Together with beeswax, a pinch of borax can help to bind creams.

Calendula Oil (Pot Marigold)
(Calendula officinalis)

Calendula oil is derived through extraction from the golden-yellow flowers of the plant. Its consistency is thick, the color yellowish.

Use calendula oil for chapped, brittle, scaly skin, for general skin care and healing, hand care, the treatment of blood effusions and bruises, the sore nipples of nursing mothers, varicose veins, and chronic abscesses. Its healing power has been known and used in ointments and tinctures throughout Europe and America for hundreds of years. Calendula is a valuable skin oil for the entire body. Its fragrance is herb-like, strong, and slightly bitter.

Clay

Clay clears the skin, stimulates circulation, and is anti-inflammatory. It is one of the best skin cleansers available, for it draws out toxins like a magnet. It also contains valuable minerals such as siliceous earth, iron, magnesium, zinc, and potassium. The minerals stored in the tissue of the body protect the tissue against loss of liquids. If there are not enough minerals present, the tissue becomes dry, tired, and sluggish.

Clay can be used as a basic substance for cleansing every type of skin, particularly in the form of masks for blemished, oily, tired, and aging skin. Warmth is created beneath the mask, the skin begins to sweat, as a result toxins, waste products, and dirt are discharged and no longer block the elimination process in and on the upper surface of the skin.

Green clay, which reduces sebaceous production, is primarily suited for oily skin; *white and brown* clay, which particularly supports detoxification and balances sebaceous production, is suitable for dry as well as oily skin, while *red* clay is used for cleansing and to maintain normal skin. *Blue* clay, which contains cobalt salts and is difficult to find, is particularly valuable for the treatment of acne and of infected, sensitive skin.

Cocoa Butter

Cocoa butter is a by-product of cocoa pressing. It is obtained from the roasted cocoa beans that are the primary ingredient in chocolate or cocoa. The light-sensitive butter is yellowish, suet-like, and has a pleasant scent. It does not irritate the skin, and since it slows the loss of moisture is primarily used as a binder and moisturizer in the production of creams.

Pure cocoa butter can be applied gently to wrinkles and furrows. It is best to use cocoa butter and lanolin together, since they complement each other. The lanolin becomes less sticky, while the cocoa butter is more easily absorbed by the skin.

Coconut Oil

This oil is made by pressing the coconut kernels. It inhibits the loss of skin moisture since it melts on the skin and is hardly absorbed. It makes the skin smooth and is a good after-sun oil. Coconut oil is used in cosmetics to give lotions and creams a smooth consistency. It can also be chemically bound with salts and used to produce soaps. The oil has the strong, typical coconut fragrance. The derivative of coconut oil makes oils hydrophile, which means that they dissolve in water (in bath oils, for example).

Distilled Water

Distilled water is absolutely pure water. The less expensive "purified water" is free of bacteria, salts, dust, and inorganic substances. Both are used for making cosmetics since tap water contains chemical additives and is not pure. However, boiled water is adequate for making shampoos and rinses.

Emulsifiers and Thickeners

Emulsifiers—substances that bind water with oil or fat—are needed to make creams, ointments, and lotions. Commercial cosmetic products mostly use chemically manufactured emulsifiers that can reduce or destroy entirely the effects of natural substances. Natural cosmetic creams, by contrast, contain natural emulsifiers such as beeswax (combined with borax), jojoba oil (which thickens at temperatures around 50°F), cocoa butter, glycerine, and lanolin or anhydrous lanolin. If the proportion of fat contained in a cream is less than 50%, an emulsifier is always necessary. The most natural emulsifier is the instruction to "shake before using." Liquids need thickeners to give them a better consistency for application to the skin or hair. Shampoos, shower gels, hand-washing gels, and lotions are best thickened with pectin (most effective), agar-agar, lecithin, or glycerine.

Flower Waters

Flower waters are created when essential oils are obtained through the steam distillation process and the water is richly saturated with the hydrophile substances of the blossoms. The resultant oils and water have a rejuvenating effect upon the skin.

The American market is most familiar with rose, lavender, and orange blossom waters. These floral waters contain skin-soothing substances that are not found in the corresponding essential oils, and are free of irritating terpenes and other hydrocarbons. Their effect is antiseptic, anti-inflammatory, cooling, and astringent. They are a basic ingredient in many of my recipes, since pure flower water is an excellent component in facial compresses and mild facial lotions.

Glycerine

This colorless syrup can be distilled either synthetically, from alcohol, or naturally, from vegetable oils. Natural glycerine has been used for hundreds of years to bind, lubricate, and dilute cosmetic mixtures, as well as being a common ingredient in soap. It is said to carry moisture to the skin, but only when a high degree of humidity is already present in the air, so that one does not actually need a moisturizer. On the other hand, it has also been maintained that glycerine robs the skin of moisture and can irritate sensitive skin.

Hazelnut Oil

Hazelnut oil is used especially in sun oils or sun-protection oils. Buy only the cold-pressed oil.

Honey

Honey is used in the preparation of creams, lotions, masks, and bath additives. The qualities of the slightly antiseptic, bacteriostatic honey are useful in products that soothe, smooth, heal, and nourish the skin. It also serves as a natural bonding agent in packs and masks. In hair lotions, honey has the effect of a setting lotion.

Honey contains about ten enzymes, one hormone (acetylcholin), inhibin (a bacteriostatic agent, similar to antibiotics), phosphate, calcium, magnesium, copper, manganese, potassium, iron, and vitamins B_2, B_6, and C. It is best to use only naturally pure, unheated honey. Honey should not be exposed to temperatures above 100°F, which will destroy its active ingredients.

Jojoba Oil

Jojoba oil is derived from a plant that grows in California, Arizona, and Mexico. It lives as long as one hundred years and thrives in the desert at temperatures as high as 122°F, without noticeable absorption of water. A waxy coating seals the entire plant, making it possible for it to thrive in such a climate by allowing no liquids to evaporate, storing what it receives in the way of rainfall, and surviving the extreme cold at night. This wax is found particularly in jojoba beans, which are harvested in amounts up to 13 pounds per bush. Jojoba oil is actually not an oil at all, then, but rather a liquid wax. It is effective only when it is not mixed with synthetic substances such as preservatives. Some commercial products use fermented jojoba flour (which is cheaper) or jojoba tincture, but both these forms lose their effectiveness in the synthetic soup to which they are added. You should therefore only use pure jojoba oil.

High-quality jojoba oil is without color or smell and therefore ideal for cosmetics. It does not become rancid and is a wonderful way to treat skin and hair. A facial oil made of jojoba oil and essential oils can be favorably compared with any expensive cream. Use jojoba oil for all facial and body oils, masks, packs, as well as the oily portion of creams and lotions. Jojoba oil is also effective against acne.

Jojoba oil is further known as an effective ingredient in shampoos, in hair treatments and packs, and in the treatment of damaged, brittle hair, hair loss, and split ends. Finally, it can be used in a hot oil treatment for the stimulation and cleansing of the scalp. The wax acts on the skin and hair just as it does on the plant: it forms a fine, protective, nongreasy film. The skin becomes silky and soft, the hair shines.

Another useful quality of jojoba oil is that it becomes firm at temperatures below 50°F. This characteristic can be taken advantage of when making natural creams that need to be kept cool: creams containing jojoba oil become very firm and not rancid in the refrigerator. The oil also emulsifies well in a cream with beeswax and borax.

Lanolin

Also called "wool grease," lanolin is obtained from the fat in sheep's wool. It is protective and beneficial coating for the skin, contributing moisture and well suited for the treatment of split or brittle hair, cracked skin on the foot, dry and raw elbows and knees, extremely dry skin, chapped and cracked hands, brittle fingernails, and the sore nipples of nursing mothers. It protects the skin particularly in winter—during winter sports when extreme cold, strong wind, or sunshine in the high mountains are present.

Since lanolin easily becomes rancid, buy only the amount needed for preparation and keep it in the refrigerator. Essential oils or vitamin E oil delay the oxidation process in homemade cosmetics. Anhydrous lanolin contains no oil, binds water, and is therefore often used as an emulsifier, base, and emollient in creams and lotions. When mixed with cocoa butter, wax, and oil, lanolin loses its stickiness. Creams to which lanolin has been added can be more easily spread and stay on the skin longer.

Studies in the United States have shown that the possibility of an allergic reaction to lanolin is around 0.01%. Even those who cannot tolerate wool against the skin can use lanolin. If lanolin does cause a reaction and thus cannot be used as an emulsifier, beeswax and borax may be substituted.

Lavender Water

see Flower Waters

Lethicin

Lethicin is a vegetable substance that can be used as an emulsifier in creams and lotions and also as a thickener in soaps and shampoos.

Milk

Milk is an inexpensive beauty aid containing vitamin A, protein, and fat. Use fresh whole milk in baths for sensitive skin, add honey for dry skin, and wheat germ for blemished skin. Whole milk can also be used instead of water in all masks since it stimulates and cares for the skin. Finally, brittle, dull hair turns shiny and soft after a milk rinse that is left in the hair for an hour.

Mineral Oil

Mineral oil is a purified light petroleum oil that cannot become rancid. Although it makes the skin smooth, it is not effective with added substances, is not dissoved by the sebaceous fat, and forms a thick protective layer that does stop the evaporation of moisture, yet "sits" on the skin like an oil slick and prevents it from breathing. Because of its nonperishability, the industry makes generous use of this oil. However, since it has no skin care effect and is inorganic, mineral oil is not used in natural cosmetics.

Moisturizer

Moisturizer is used to reduce the loss of skin moisture. Its effect is short-lived; it is best applied regularly in lotion or cream form to the damp skin after bathing or showering. It affects the surface layer of the skin only, causing it to swell. The skin then becomes soft and smooth. The most effective moisturizers are vegetable oils, lanolin, cocoa butter, and glycerine.

Mineral oils are often added liberally to commercial moisturizers or lotions, yet they are not organic substances and cannot be absorbed. (See "Mineral Oil.")

Olive Oil

This oil, obtained by pressing ripe olives, has a spicy scent and is greenish-yellow. A valuable oil for skin care, olive oil has been used for centuries as a cosmetic and food by the peoples of the Mediterranean region. Use only the olive oil of the first cold pressing ("extra vierge") for creams, lotions, hair treatments and ointments. It is very beneficial for dry, damaged, or split hair.

Orange Blossom Water

see Flower Waters

Peanut Oil

Peanut oil, made by pressing peanuts, is absorbed very well by the skin, is rich in vitamin E and unsaturated fatty acids, and hardly ever becomes rancid. Yet it is seldom used in cosmetics because of its heavy odor.

Pectin

Pectin, a natural thickener, is found in the roots, stems, and fruit of all plants. It is used in cosmetics to thicken gels, lotions, and creams.

Petroleum Jelly

A mineral fat, this viscous, transparent, odorless mass is widely available commercially. Petroleum jelly does not penetrate the skin and in this respect does not affect it, but is suitable for use in healing ointments for wounds and protective creams. An excellent natural substitute is jojoba ointment.

Polysorbates
(Tween 60, 80)

These synthetic emulsifiers (substances that make oils water-soluble) are used to manufacture many commercial products (creams, lotions, gels). Tween does not irritate the skin, is clear, oily, and available in liquid form. Although the FDA has approved its use as an emulsifier in cosmetics and has classified it as "suitable for use in foods," some caution seems warranted, since many substances have been "approved," only later to be proven injurious to health. One teaspoon of Tween to 16 ounces of vegetable oil is sufficient to dissolve the bath oil in water. Essential oils can also be made water-soluble with Tween. A natural substitute is coconut derivative.

Rosewater

see Flower Waters

Sesame Oil

Sesame oil, obtained by pressing sesame seeds, blocks about 30% of the sun's UV rays and can therefore be used as a sun protection oil. It is yellowish and odorless. Since it easily becomes rancid, it must be stored in a cool place. Sesame oil should be mixed with a vegetable oil that inhibits oxidation (wheat-germ oil, jojoba oil) or an essential oil such as benzoin. If possible, use only cold-pressed oil.

Soaps

Homemade soap, shampoo, or liquid shower soap can be made using white soft soap, curd soap, pure soap, or natural soaps (olive, rose, lavender, almond soap) as a base. A few drops of essential oils will provide a personalized fragrance.

Soy Oil

Made from ripe, fresh soy beans, soy oil is yellow, odorless, and very thin. It contains many vitamins and is suitable for skin care.

However, it may trigger an allergic reaction in some cases in the form of skin eruptions, so test it first on a small area. Use only cold-pressed oil when possible.

Sweet Almond Oil

This high-quality vegetable oil is well absorbed by the skin and thus can help in the penetration of essential oils into the skin. Sweet almond oil, derived from the ripe seeds or sweet almonds of the almond tree, smooths and maintains the skin. Yellowish in color and odorless, it is ideal for making skin-care oils and creams. If possible, use only cold-pressed oils.

Vinegar

Apple cider vinegar is an inexpensive beauty aid that can be mixed with essential oils to rinse calcium remnants and soap residue from the hair. Vinegar is also helpful against dandruff. Added to the bath, it cleans greasy, blemished skin. Facial skin is particularly well cleansed by a mixture of vinegar, pure water, and a few drops of peppermint or juniper. It is also recommended for aftershave lotions. Wine vinegar has the same effect and also promotes circulation.

Wheat Bran

This by-product of flour production is valued for its soothing, anti-inflammatory, and healing qualities. Bran contains vitamin B_6, which is important for cell renewal. Its main use is in skin care baths and for masks. Wheat bran cleanses the skin and makes it soft.

Wheat Germ Oil

Because this golden-yellow to brownish oil smells strongly of wheat, its possibilities for use in cosmetics are limited. Wheat germ oil contains many vitamins, particularly vitamin E, as well as carotene, vegetable lecithin, and unsaturated fatty acids, and rarely turns rancid. It can be added to other oils, to extend their stability.

Wheat germ oil is also a valuable additive to skin oils. It smooths the skin, prevents the loss of moisture, and benefits the cells. Finally, it treats and strengthens dry and split hair when massaged into the split ends and left on for about 15 minutes before washing the hair. As with all other vegetable oils, only cold-pressed oil should be used.

Witch Hazel

Witch hazel is an alcoholic extract from the leaves, flowers, and bark of the hamamelis tree. It is used in cosmetics because of its healing, toning, anti-inflammatory, and astringent qualities. Pure witch hazel solution is a good skin tonic for mature, tired, sluggish, oily, blemished, and infected skin or scalp. It is also particularly recommended as an aftershave lotion.

Yogurt

Yogurt contains lactic acid and can be used externally in packs and masks for large-pored, oily, and blemished skin. Eating yogurt is the best natural way to care for the skin.

Purchasing Ready-made Natural Cosmetics

Some readers may prefer buying ready-made natural cosmetic products to making their own. The manufacturers of such products are rare and the products relatively expensive, but they are preferable to those produced by the large cosmetic manufacturers. Because of their limited shelf life (up to six months), fresh cosmetic products must be replaced at regular intervals. Their price naturally depends on the demand. When small amounts are made labor-intensively, they cannot compete with the mass-produced commercial cosmetics.

Natural and fresh cosmetics are found in natural cosmetic stores, health food stores, and natural food stores. These products are almost—but not quite—equal in value to homemade natural cosmetics.

Making Natural Cosmetics at Home

You will need the following equipment:

- 2 double boilers (or heatproof bowls that may be placed over a pot of boiling water)
- a large bowl made of heatproof glass
- a small heat-resistant glass or ceramic jar for warming ingredients
- a wooden spoon
- a clear measuring cup
- plastic containers or beakers
- a thermometer with readings to 200°F
- a hand mixer
- several stainless steel wisks
- a funnel
- a small (postage) scale
- empty glass or porcelain jars for creams, dark (amber-colored) bottles for toners and body and facial oils
- labels and a waterproof felt-tip pen
- a cosmetic brush for applying liquid masks
- cotton balls to apply and remove facial oils
- a shower cap for hair treatments

Supply sources for many of the basic ingredients and essential oils are natural cosmetic stores, health food stores, herb shops, and natural food stores. These stores may also carry good basic shampoos, creams, lotions, toners, and so on, which can be made fragrant and effective by adding a few drops of essential oil. Since only natural, pure oils should be used, I recommend that you look for a store with trained personnel.

Other ingredients (lanolin, cocoa butter, lecithin, glycerine, alum, clay, etc.) can be obtained in pharmacies. Pectin can usually be found in grocery stores or large natural-food stores in the baking or home-canning supply section.

Essential oils can also be purchased directly from the suppliers. Some manufacturers and suppliers guarantee that their essential oils are natural and pure. It is always worthwhile to compare prices, especially for essential oils. Those which cost considerably less than the average price may be synthetic, stretched, or perfume oils. These oils are not suitable for cosmetics.

Preparation:

When hand-mixing—the best method for even, quick mixing of a mass—use a mixing whisk to prevent splattering. Keep a second, clean mixing whisk ready for the next blend. When weighing, always use the same container, subtracting its weight from the entire weight. That way the weight does not need to be recalculated every time. A letter scale with an adjustable screw works well for this purpose, since you can set the pointer at zero after putting the measuring container on it.

As in cooking, do not be overanxious about precision in measuring, and do not despair if the result does not immediately preent the desired consistency. A teaspoon is not always a teaspoon! If a cream or lotion is not firm or creamy enough on the first attempt, simply experiment with the recipe's proportions until you are satisfied. There is a vast range of essential oils, emulsifiers and vegetable oils from which to choose.

It is very important in water-in-oil emulsions to add the water slowly until the cream has attained the desired consistency. Every emulsion becomes harder after cooling. Allow time for each process: do not try to shorten the cooling time, for example, by putting the mixture in a cold water bath or in the refrigerator.

Cleanliness in making and filling the cosmetics is imperative since natural cosmetics do not tolerate bacteria or germs. All mixtures are to be warmed in a double boiler (that is over—not in—hot water); *never* heat them directly over a flame.

I recommend that you buy all the ingredients only in the amounts needed for the next preparation, and keep them in the refrigerator. Essential oils and vegetable oils must be stored in amber-colored bottles. Citrus oils will not keep longer than six months. Creams, lotions, masks, and so on should be stored in the refrigerator in clay, porcelain, or glass containers since plastic can lead to chemical reactions with the essential oils. On the basis of my own experience, I cannot recommend "food-safe" plastic containers either.

Essential oils preserve themselves. To support this process, however, the anti-oxidation properties of vegetable oils can be added. Wheat-germ oil (added in a proportion of about 10%) will prevent skin care and bath oils will from becoming rancid. A few drops of benzoin oil also extend the shelf life of a mixture. This, of course, does not provide the same long-term protection for homemade cosmetics as can be obtained with synthetic preservatives. You should therefore only make as much as you can use within the next two to three months. The shelf life of any product depends upon various factors: which substances you use, whether anti-oxidants are among the ingredients, how fresh the substances are when you use them, and if they have been stored in a cool place.

After preparation, clean all equipment in boiling water or at least wash them out with hot soapy water, rinse them well, and dry them. It is best to use these utensils only for making cosmetics and not prepare or store food in them at other times.

4 Skin Care

Structure and Functions of the Skin

Our skin is a constantly changing environment made up of many different layers. Viewed under a microscope, the surface of the skin does not look smooth and symmetrical at all. There are hills, mountains, and valleys. Liquids flow through small openings to the surface. Hair, resembling swamp grass, grows everywhere. Germs and bacteria frisk around, keeping the environment clean, healthy, and in equilibrium—a balanced system of fauna and flora. Like our earth, the microcosm of the skin can become unbalanced by overexposure to toxins, ultraviolet rays, and dirt. A smooth and harmonic functioning also requires the appropriate nourishment in the form of protein, minerals, vitamins, and liquids.

Our skin changes constantly, from the stage of infancy, when it is soft, tender, supple, and wrinkle-free, to the years of maturity, when it becomes harder and drier because of changes in the amount of collagen, and when wrinkles form. These are the most obvious and unavoidable changes. The condition of the skin is also changed by environmental influences, nutrition, illness, age, and emotional states. Stress, nervousness, fear, frustration, aggravation, love, satisfaction, and joy are more clearly expressed in the skin as a mirror of our inner lives than is commonly assumed. Various skin disturbances can indicate that the emotional world is not in balance. Most obviously, our feelings are shown within seconds by the skin when we blush, grow pale, or start to sweat.

The skin, which is made up of a number of layers, represents about 20% of the body weight and has a surface of about 2.1 square yards for a person of average size. It transports 42 gallons of blood and 1–3 gallons of water in 24 hours.

The outermost, visible skin layer, the epidermis, is about 0.05 inches thick, and is primarily composed of seven layers of dead epidermal cells. This horn-like zone, which seals the skin, is so dense that only simple molecules can penetrate it. Older skin retains only two to three layers, which can no longer bind enough moisture to keep from drying out. Since circulation also weakens with aging, the fatty proportion of the lower tissue also decreases, causing wrinkles and marked facial lines to occur.

Metochromatic granules, the pigments which contain melanin, are stored in the epidermis. They determine our skin coloring. The more pigments there are and the higher they are in the horny zone, the darker the skin will be. The horny zone is located above the stratum lucidum and a fine layer of keratin, which together create the actual protective covering of the skin. The lowest layer of the epidermis is the germinative layer, where new skin cells are constantly being formed, forcing the old skin cells outward or upward into the horny zone. These uppermost cells then peel off through washing or rub off against clothing and sheets. A period of four weeks usually goes by from the formation of a new skin cell to its peeling off, so that the skin renews itself every month. If the skin does not peel off normally, it will become hard and sluggish.

The next layer, the dermis (also called corium or cutis), contains the elastic filaments that make up the connective tissue. The connective tissue substance, the matrix, is tender and gelatinous in small children, but changes into the firm, robust substance known as collagen in the course of life.

A further main component of the connective tissue is elastin. As we age, cross-connections occur between the filaments of the connective tissue that were originally parallel to each other, and bind the water in the spaces between them, like a coarsely-knit sweater that initially leaves much room for air to circulate, but that becomes more and more matted through frequent laundering in hot water. Every cell of the body lies bedded in this substance in such a manner.

Not only advancing age, but also environmental toxins, poor nutrition, lack of oxygen, weak circulation, hormonal changes, stress, emotional burdens, and inherited factors change this basic substance. The more difficult we feel life to be and the more we build defensive mental and emotional walls against our environment, the more the collagen hardens. As it solidifies, the air space is reduced. The skin becomes less able to take up moisture, and the collagen can even be eaten away. The subcutis then begins to wrinkle and shrink. Since the epidermis itself does not change, it responds by becoming wrinkled and furrowed.

Collagen and elastin are renewed only with outside help—a promise held out by certain collagen-containing cosmetic products, despite the fact that the large molecules involved cannot penetrate the horny zone. A treatment with vitamin A acid, which supposedly forms new collagen, has also been recommended. However, this treatment does have side effects and is costly—and it has not been absolutely demonstrated that new collagen is actually created.

By comparison, the renewal process of the skin cells can be stimulated with essential oils. Further natural preventive measures against rapid skin aging are foods rich in minerals and vitamins (vitamins C, E), exercise, increased oxygen supply, avoidance of nicotine and caffeine, moderate sun exposure, and an adequate intake of fluids. Finally, a harmonic, stress-free lifestyle will help to maintain the condition of the skin and connective tissue and counteract the rapid cross-linkage or dismantling of collagen.

The dermis also contains the blood vessels that carry oxygen and nutrients from the body to the upper skin layers, lymph ducts, pigment cells, sweat glands (about 650 per square inch), sebaceous glands, nerve fibers, and the hair roots (hair follicles). The sweat glands eliminate toxic substances and waste products, and regulate the body temperature. The perspiration they secrete continually is made almost entirely of water. In addition, there are traces of salt, carbohydrates, protein, and oil. An adult has about three million sweat glands, one third of which are located in the pubic hair, underarm, and head areas, where the perspiration mixes with bacteria and determines the body's scent. The amount of perspiration—and the body scent it conveys—increases in the evening (a time when the body temperature rises as well).

The sebaceous glands, appendages found next to each hair shaft, provide the hair with sebum, making it smooth, dirt-resistant, and protected against drying out. They also contribute to the oil content of the skin. Some 300,000 of these sebaceous glands produce about 0.07 ounces of sebum daily. When the ends of the sebaceous glands are plugged, pimples, pustules, blackheads, and infections form. An overproduction of sebum causes oily skin and promotes acne. This activity is provoked by hormonal changes during puberty or during the menstrual cycle, by high dosages of estrogen, or by foods that contain or stimulate estrogen. When too little sebum is produced, on the other hand, the skin is dry and scaly. Geranium, frankincense, and ylang-ylang have a balancing effect on sebum production. Bergamot, lavender, juniper, and lemon have a reductive effect; carrot seed has a stimulating effect. Perspiration, skin scales, and sebum together build the acid mantle of the skin, the "ozone layer" that protects us from deadly radiation.

The five million nerve cells of the skin with their ten billion sensors signal every change in temperature, every touch, every surface condition, every instance of pain or itching through the nervous system to the brain, which then causes the body to respond. These nerve cells are particularly concentrated in the lips and fingertips, so that touch is felt as very intense in these areas.

The bottommost skin layer, the subcutis or hypodermis, is a

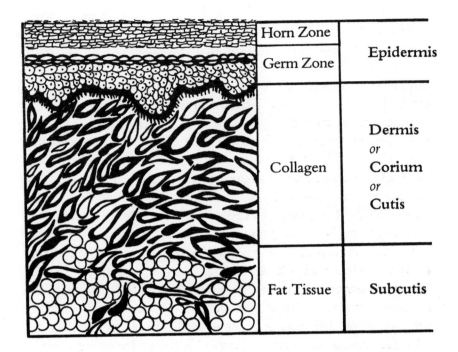

		Epidermis
	Horn Zone	Epidermis
	Germ Zone	
	Collagen	Dermis *or* Corium *or* Cutis
	Fat Tissue	Subcutis

Figure 1: The three layers of skin

seamless continuation of the dermis, consisting of loose connective tissue, the fatty tissue, lymph ducts, and blood vessels. If the tissue becomes hard, the skin layers around it can no longer properly move back and forth: the skin loses its elasticity. This layer is mainly "padding," storing up to 44 pounds of fat.

The skin has many tasks, the most important of which is to protect the body against penetration by dirt, germs, and foreign substances such as acids, alkalines, and toxic substances. It forms an acid mantle that eliminates germs through acidic perspiration, scales of cornified epithelium, and sebum as well as through secreted carbon dioxide.

The skin is normally host to some twenty billion beneficial germs in the pubic and underarm areas. These germs are destroyed through

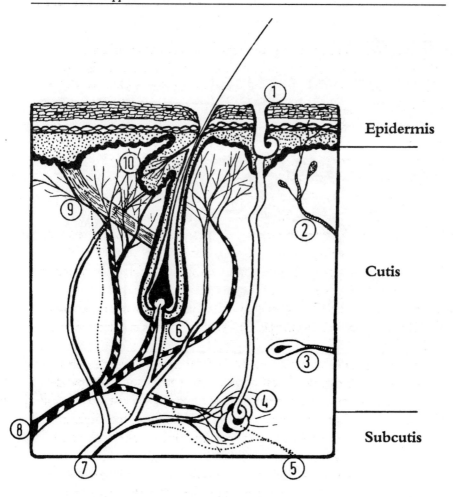

Epidermis

Cutis

Subcutis

1 = sweat pore
2 = nerve ending for hot
    and cold
3 = nerve ending for pain
4 = sweat gland
5 = autonomous nerve system

6 = hair, hair shaft,
    hair root
7 = artery
8 = vein
9 = erector pili muscl
10 = sebaceous gland

Figure 2: Cross section of the skin through three layers

aggressive substances such as wash-active substances (tensides), synthetic soaps, strong preservatives or chemical dyes, as well as by bathing or showering too long and too hot, or through stress. Other germs can then spread. In general the acid mantle builds up again twenty minutes after bathing or washing, but it loses its effectiveness when constantly exposed to the aggressive substances contained in many synthetic creams, lotions, and washing agents.

The acid mantle of the skin has a pH value of 4.8–6. (The pH value [pH = potentia hydrogenii = hydrogen ion concentration] gives the acid or alkaline content of a substance: when the pH value is less than 7, the substance is acidic; when it is more than 7, the substance is alkaline and no longer corresponds to that of the acid mantle. A substance is said to have a neutral pH value when it is between 6.5–7.) Soaps, particularly synthetic soaps, are mostly alkaline. You should therefore only wash yourself with those soaps and shampoos having a neutral pH value, which is most beneficial for the skin.

Our skin regulates temperature of its fatty layers through perspiration and also controls body temperature by narrowing or expanding the blood vessels, thereby protecting us from excessive heat and cold. When it is hot, the body withdraws heat from the organism through perspiration and by expanding the blood vessels. When it is cold, the blood vessels narrow, the sebaceous glands secrete sebum, which spreads like a protective coating over the dermis, and the sweat glands secrete less perspiration. The skin gives off 70% of the warmth created by metabolism. This is why people experience cold more readily when the metabolism is sluggish and the diet is lacking in nutrients.

The skin also protects us from excessive solar radiation. Longer exposure to the sun leads to the increased formation of melanin, the pigment that gives our skin its actual color. The more these pigments in the skin are stimulated through ultraviolet radiation or warmth, the darker the skin becomes. Our natural protection against ultraviolet radiation has a limited effect, however. When the skin becomes overtaxed, the result is a sunburn.

The skin can store up to 44 pounds of fat and up to 22 pounds of water. It regulates 20% of the body's water elimination through perspiration and together with the kidneys tackles the task of toxic substance disposal. If the kidneys do not function as they should, the skin must take on their work as well; it is then overtaxed. Through the skin's respiration, we eliminate about 2 pints of liquid daily, which must then be replaced.

The skin receives oxygen and carbon dioxide from the air and eliminates them by the same means. Only certain substances can penetrate the skin. Among them are fat-soluble materials (e.g., certain hormones), lipoid-soluble substances, gases, phenol derivative, and essential oils. It is unclear, and there is cause to doubt, whether it can absorb collagen, elastin, and synthetic vitamins.

The production of vitamin D is another of the skin's important tasks. This function is related to the amount of sunshine available and therefore reduced in winter. Finally, the skin forms a callous layer of keratin in certain spots in order to protect the body—for example, the areas on the insides of the hands and the foot soles which are about 0.18 inches thick. The uppermost skin layer also has the effect of a light callus in order to protect us against solar radiation.

The condition and functions of the skin are clearly impaired by various situations and substances. Any of the following elements can prevent the skin from fulfilling its vital functions:

- nutritional starvation (foods lacking in vitamins and minerals)
- oxygen deficiency (closed, overheated rooms)
- nicotine
- excessive ultraviolet radiation
- air pollution
- hard, impure tap water
- swimming in chlorinated water
- occupational contact with acids and lyes
- skin care agents with synthetic substances, aggressive wash agents in soaps, shampoos, bath additives, shower gels
- medication

- excessive use of synthetic cosmetic products
- emotional influences such as stress, nervousness, aggravation, sorrow, or fear
- hard physical work in the sun, wind, and rain
- loss of skin moisture through inadequate care

Awareness of and attention to these potential problem areas can help to avert the need for an extensive skin care program.

Skin Types: Characteristics and Care with Essential Oils

Normal Skin

Normal skin is completely healthy. In youth it is smooth, fine-pored, and soft; with age it becomes dry, wrinkled, and marked with the so-called "age spots." Between these two normal conditions there are short periods of changes and irritations of the normal skin because of hormonal changes, illness, psychic problems, and so on, from which few of us are exempted in life.

Normal skin needs no extensive special care. It can be treated simply with a mild cleansing lotion, water, and a mild fat-containing, pH neutral soap, a moisturizing lotion for the body, a facial lotion, a light, nongreasy day cream, and possibly a night cream containing vegetable oils. Some vinegar should be added to the bath water, which is generally too hard for all skin types. Suitable essential oils for the care of normal skin are bergamot, Roman chamomile, lavender, geranium, neroli, rose, rosewood, and cedarwood.

Oily Skin

Oily skin is thick and tends to form pimples and blackheads. The sebaceous glands produce too much sebum, and the fatty tissue under the epidermis is very thick. Too much fat can indicate a high estrogen level. The pores of the skin are often clogged, making it necessary to clean the skin thoroughly on a regular basis.

Basil, camphor, peppermint, juniper, thyme, sage, lemon, and tea tree, mixed with witch hazel water or a vegetable oil, are best for oily skin. Alcohol should not be used, since it initially dries out the skin but then stimulates the production of sebum even more. Camphor, sage, and thyme penetrate deeply into the skin, cleanse it, contract the pores, stimulate the skin functions, and have an antiseptic effect. These oils are particularly useful for inflamed areas. Compresses and facial steam baths prepared with these three essences are very effective.

Pimples and blackheads can be treated with tea tree, lemon, or lavender. Use the pure oils, but only on the blemished spots. For basic skin care, I recommend a moisturizing cream with jojoba oil and bergamot or lavender since both oils reduce or balance the production of sebum.

Although it may sound like a contradiction, oily skin can be treated successfully with vegetable oils, which actually allow the sebum to drain gently. Vegetable oils can also be used in pure form as facial oil. Add the following essential oils to creams or lotions: geranium, camphor (sparingly), rosemary, rose, sandalwood, juniper, frankincense, ylang-ylang, cedarwood, cypress, and lemon.

A night cream should only be applied to the skin on alternate nights. Skin that is inflamed should be treated it with jojoba oil (facial oil) or witch hazel lotion (facial lotion), both combined with an anti-inflammatory oil such as geranium, blue chamomile, lavender, myrrh, peppermint, or rose.

Dry Skin

Dry skin is characterized by a lack of fat or moisture caused by inadequate production of the sebaceous glands. In such cases the acid equilibrium is out of balance and cannot be restored by the external application of water. Water cannot penetrate the skin, and in fact even more moisture is taken from the surface of the skin through evaporation when water is applied.

This skin type should avoid eau de cologne perfumes and cosmetics with alcohol. Moisturizing creams and lotions containing oil are the best method to prevent loss of moisture, especially after bathing or showering. High-quality vegetable oils with essential oils are most appropriate for this purpose. Avoid hot facial steam baths and facial masks, which strongly stimulate circulation, and apply lukewarm compresses instead. Use only little or no soap to cleanse dry skin, since it strips the skin of fat; water should be soft and not too hot when showering or bathing. I very much recommend the use of a fatty liquid soap or washing gel. Again, hard water can be softened by adding a few tablespoons of vinegar.

It is best to cleanse the face with a cleansing oil (hazelnut oil or almond oil mixed with a few drops of essential oils). The cream or facial oil necessary for dry skin care should contain either sweet almond oil, olive oil, or avocado oil, and should always include some wheat germ oil as well. The sebaceous glands are stimulated to stronger, more balanced production by special essential oils such as geranium, carrot seed, frankincense, and ylang-ylang.

Dry skin is more prone to forming wrinkles than any other skin type. The appropriate spots therefore have to be intensively treated with pure warm almond oil, wheat germ oil, or cocoa butter. However, this treatment only works on the upper layer and cannot influence the dry tissue. The following essential oils are useful for the general care of dry skin: geranium, carrot seed, Roman chamomile, lavender, jasmine, orange, rose, rosewood, sandalwood, frankincense, ylang-ylang, and cedarwood.

Mixed Skin

The mixed skin type—which is not to be confused with seborrhea—consists of two skin types, dry and oily skin. On the face, for example, there are oily areas as well as dry areas. If we come to the conclusion that each area needs a different type of treatment, then we would have to make two different kinds of cosmetics and treat both areas separately—a complicated program that we can dispense with by substituting a nongreasy skin oil (jojoba oil) and essential oils that balance the production of sebum.

In the oily areas, pimples and blackheads often form. Naturally they should be treated not with fatty creams but rather with jojoba oil and lavender, tea tree and lemon. The dry areas should additionally be treated (as for dry skin) extensively with warm almond oil, wheat germ oil, cocoa butter, and bergamot. Both areas can be treated together with Roman chamomile, rose, bergamot, and/or lavender, as well as witch hazel solution and jojoba oil.

Mature Skin

Aging or mature skin is characterized by moisture loss and advanced collagen cross-linkage, which is shown in wrinkles or facial lines. Sagging skin is a normal occurrence in the aging process. However, anyone who has this kind of skin at age 30 will be justifiably concerned. Before beginning an extensive skin care program, critical consideration should be given to such factors as nutrition; the use of alcohol, nicotine, and caffeine; exposure to fresh air and exercise; mental and emotional pressures as well as daily stress. Reduction of stress is guaranteed to bring about an improvement in the skin condition even without any special cosmetics.

To support mature skin, give it moisture and oxygen. Packs or hot compresses are suitable for this purpose. Regular use of facial scrubs will loosen hardened places in the skin by stimulating lymph flow and circulation, so that waste products are removed more quickly, nutrients are transmitted to the cells, and the cells themselves are renewed and/or peel in a normal rhythm.

An intensive cleansing with toning oils at regular intervals is very important for mature skin. The purpose of skin care is always to activate the skin. This can also be achieved through a gentle facial massage or a strong scalp massage, in addition to using the appropriate essential oils. Avocado oil, jojoba oil, and wheat germ oil should be used when making cosmetics for mature skin. The rejuvenating oils of neroli and lavender will serve well here. The following oils are suitable for the care of mature skin: carrot seed, cypress, frankincense, fennel, myrrh, orange, patchouli, rose, sandalwood, and vetiver. Bergamot, geranium, and jasmine will stimulate or balance sebaceous gland production when the skin is too dry.

Blemished Skin

Pimples and blackheads that are characteristic of blemished skin can form, as with other skin irregularities, through inadequate cleansing, air pollution, poor nutrition, change of climate, poor digestion, use of nicotine, caffeine, medication, and emotional problems.

Minor spots can be dabbed with undiluted lavender, lemon, or tea tree. After a steam bath, carefully squeeze the pimples and put some pure alcohol or tea tree on them. Very impure skin can be treated with warm compresses using the recommended essential oils as well as parsley. Apply a weekly cleansing mask with lavender, tea tree, and thyme (sparingly), or with sage (sparingly), parsley, and rosemary. These mixtures are antiseptic, stimulate skin function, cleanse the skin, and absorb inflammations.

Facial skin is best treated with oils, creams, or lotions containing jojoba oil with lavender and tea tree and lemon. These oils are antiseptic and cleansing. If blemished skin is also oily, use bergamot to counteract the overproduction of sebum.

Wrinkles and Facial Lines

In an age in which the media proclaim that youth is the indispensable prerequisite for success, well-being, recognition, and popularity, it has become increasingly difficult to live with wrinkles, whether they are caused by environmental factors, poor life care habits, or the tension and hardening that leave their mark on the face as "worry wrinkles." Yet another reason for wrinkles is fre-

quent laughter, which causes "laugh lines." In fact, laughter uses far
fewer facial muscles than do expressions of aggravation, anger, or
fear. We need the release of periodic laughter and tears to be
balanced, complete human beings. (Think about it for a moment:
Would we actually want to spend our adult years in the company
of wrinkle-free people who never laughed or cried?) The whole
fuss about wrinkles originates from the cosmetic industry, its sole
long-term beneficiary.

If your facial lines bother you, dab them lightly with pure cocoa
butter, warm jojoba oil, almond oil, or wheat germ oil. A wrinkle
cream can also be made using carrot seed and frankincense or
neroli. Underlying muscle tension can be relieved with a facial
massage or Shiatsu massage (see pages 146–150).

Sensitive Skin

Delicate, sensitive skin reacts more strongly than any other skin
type to many substances in medication and synthetic cosmetics, to
dirt, toxins, weather factors, hormonal changes, stress, psychological
problems, dietary errors, inadequate exercise, lack of oxygen, and
sluggish metabolism. People who are generally not robust usually
have to deal with sensitive skin. Symptomatic are intense stress
conditions and nervous agitation, although the underlying causes
are often difficult to pin down precisely.

In the case of sensitive skin, it is essential to note exactly
when the irritations occur. The symptoms are skin reddening,
inflammations, dermatitis (which can also be a result of premenstrual syndrome), and itching. Care of such skin should
follow a simple principle: be sure the treatment is not too hot,
too prolonged, too oily, too strong, or too frequent This
principle applies particularly to the use of soap and shampoo. It
is best to either use none at all or a soap that is utterly mild,
fatty, and free of alkaline. A fine fragrance such as jasmine,
rose, or orange should be used for this type of skin, along with
a soothing oil such as Roman chamomile. The most effective

method can only be found through experimenting. A change in living and eating habits can often bring about positive results.

Tired Skin

As a result of mechanical influences, poor nutrition, lack of oxygen, lack of sleep, change of climate, intensive nightlife, and the misuse of alcohol, nicotine, and other drugs, the skin often becomes pale and tired. In addition to appropriate care, this type of skin needs stimulation to recover.

Compresses, steam baths, masks, and facial lotions prepared with clary sage, orange, parsley, sage (used sparingly), rosemary, or lemon activate the skin and restore skin color. Some apple cider vinegar added to the facial lotion and a strong scalp massage can work wonders.

Baby Skin

Baby skin is very sensitive and not yet fully developed. It doesn't yet have the resistance of mature skin and the acid mantle does not yet function like that of an adult. This skin and its irritations or inflammations (sore parts of the body, chapped facial skin, scaly rash, cradle cap) should be treated not with mineral oil, which most baby oils contain, but rather with jojoba oil, almond oil, and a few drops of essential oils. Please be certain that their proportion in skin oils and creams as well as in skin care baths are limited to a few drops only to avoid irritation. A skin care bath scented with tangerine or orange, for example, will delight any child. Skin care oils for the skin of babies and children are Roman chamomile and rose. These oils have a mild, healing effect and are relaxing as well.

The table on the following page summarizes the skin care applications of the oils for the skin types discussed here and provides additional guidance for their treatment.

Oils Categorized by Skin Type	baby skin	blemished skin	chapped skin	clogged skin	dehydrated skin	dry skin	facial lines	flabby skin	general skin care	inflammed skin, chronic	mature skin	mixed skin	normal skin	oily skin	sensitive skin	tired skin	hydrated skin	wrinkles
Anise							•	•										•
Basil				•														
Bergamot									•				•	•	•			
Camphor							•					•						
Carrot Seed			•				•											•
Cedarwood						•			•					•	•		•	
Chamomile, Roman	•					•							•	•		•		
Clary Sage	•							•	•							•	•	
Cypress							•				•			•		•	•	•
Fennel							•	•			•							•
Frankincense							•			•				•				•
Geranium					•	•			•		•			•	•			
Immortelle			•															
Jasmine						•			•						•			
Juniper				•										•				
Lavender		•	•			•			•		•	•	•	•				
Lemon		•	•						•					•		•		
Melissa									•									
Myrrh											•							
Myrtle									•									
Neroli								•	•				•					•
Orange	•								•					•	•	•		
Parsley						•						•						
Patchouli		•							•		•						•	
Peppermint		•												•				
Rose	•			•		•			•		•		•	•	•			
Rosemary		•												•		•		
Rosewood						•			•				•					
Sage		•						•								•		
Sandalwood			•		•	•			•	•				•				
Tea Tree		•																
Thyme		•																
Vetiver												•						
Ylang-ylang						•			•					•				

Treating Irritations and Diseases of the Skin and Tissue with Essential Oils

Dermatologists, tell us that one third of all skin diseases are psycho-somatic in origin. Further factors are environmental influences, inadequate or improper skin care, synthetic skin care substances, and aggressive cleansing agents.

Seborrhea

Seborrhea is a common condition that manifests itself in two contrasting skin pictures: either a very oily or a very dry skin with massive scale formation. Both skin reactions are the result of a metabolism that has become unbalanced because of hormonal irregularity (cyclic disturbances in women), digestive problems, improper eating habits, stress, and other influences.

Oily seborrhea is the result of an overactive sebaceous gland, an inherited condition whereby too much sebum is produced and the sebaceous fat composition is imbalanced. The skin becomes exces-sively oily, the acid equilibrium is disturbed, the way is paved for infections and acne, the pores become expanded with excess sebum, and the skin takes on an oily shine. The production of sebum must then be inhibited, with the help of essential oils, for example.

As in the case of oily skin, the seborrhic spots should be thor-oughly cleansed with camphor (sparingly), juniper, lemon, and peppermint, but not dried out forcibly with alcohol. The cleansing substance may contain alcohol only in very limited dosages, since intense drying stimulates the sebaceous glands even more afterward, and the skin becomes even oilier. A suitable skin oil (or cream) should be made of anti-inflammatory and acne-healing oils (lavender, tea tree, lemon) together with oils that decrease the functioning of the oil glands (bergamot, geranium, lemon, ylang-ylang). If necessary, minor inflammations and acne should be treated locally with a special blend of oils.

Dry seborrhea begins with a simultaneous increase in production and lowered rate of elimination of epidermal scales. This condition leads to clogging of the excretory ducts and an increased production of sebum, while the hardening process of the epidermis is accelerated and the cells die more quickly and are deposited on the surface of the skin together with the sebum. As a result, blackheads form and the skin is dry, scaly, and sallow. This sallowness is caused in part by inadequate peripheral circulation (a condition that often prevails in this type of skin). As in the case of dry skin, it is advisable to open the excretory ducts with masks, rubbing masks, and warm, damp compresses. Skin oils should contain at least 5% vitamin E oil, and include lavender and bergamot. As a supplement, take vitamin A orally or eat the appropriate vitamin-rich foods.

Acne

Acne is a disease of the skin and primarily occurs during puberty as teenage acne or as menstrual acne up to the time of menopause. It is related to hormonal changes at the onset of gonad or ovary function or the menstrual cycle. Acne occasionally also occurs at the start of menopause in women. As already mentioned, pills containing large amounts of estrogen or food with a large proportion of estrogen substances also cause or promote acne. Inadequate cleansing of the skin, improper nutrition (animal fats, sugar, coffee, tea, spices, cream), poor digestion, change of climate (travel), inherited skin sensitivity, psychological stress, nicotine, alcohol, and medications can also produce or encourage acne.

In young people, a number of causes often work together to trigger acne: the body begins to release sexual hormones, which leads to hormonal change throughout the body. Sweat glands and pores are stimulated, more fat is suddenly produced, and perspiration and fat are scented through the sexual hormones. At the same time, young people are often exposed to alcohol, cigarettes, and drugs, all of which have adverse effects on the skin.

Other contributing factors are psychological problems such as fear, social, or school-related stress, and so on. The appearance of the skin is affected, creating additional stress, so that treatment means healing not only the acne but also the frame of mind (through the use of soothing, antidepressive fragrances, for example). Stress can also be observed in women whose skin condition becomes worse every month or who constantly suffer because of acne.

Acne is a disease of the sebaceous glands and hair follicles, involving an overproduction of sebum and the development of bacteria in the sebaceous glands. The surplus sebum cannot flow off quickly enough because of the excessively thick openings, which then become clogged. Yellow sebum forms and gradually becomes black on exposure to the air, forming blackheads (comedos). The sebaceous glands continue to produce sebum. The pressure of excessive sebum in the connective tissue increases and creates inflammations, abscesses, knots, or pimples.

In the case of menstrual acne, premenstrual water retention contributes to the physical tension. All of the various forms of acne can leave ugly scars behind.

The treatment of acne aims to heal infection, stimulate lymph flow and blood circulation, and reduce the amount of sebum as well as to reduce the waste products and toxic substances deposited in the skin. Attention must be given to proper nutrition (vitamin E, B_6) and sufficient exercise, fresh air, and sun. The skin itself can be treated with camphor (sparingly), peppermint and/or juniper. Frequent masks prepared with zinc and sulfur are helpful. The masks should contain anti-inflammatory and cleansing essential oils such as cajeput, camphor (sparingly), niauoli, or tea tree. Peeling masks are used to remove the upper layer of the skin so that pimples are opened, the pores cleansed, and the circulation stimulated, allowing the sebum to flow out. A skin oil for everyday use in such cases should contain bergamot, camphor, geranium, lavender, and tea tree. Together these oils have a soothing, antibacterial, antiseptic, astringent, rejuvenating, healing, and regulating effect on sebum production. The antidepressive scent of bergamot will lighten the mood. The oil or cream should contain jojoba oil and at least 10% wheat germ oil and/or vitamin E oil. Other effective oils are Roman chamomile, rose, and patchouli. Use warm compresses made of these oils regularly. In the case of intense inflammation, tea tree and lavender can also be applied locally in undiluted form. As an alternative, a special acne ointment may be made containing 3% essential oil (see page 135).

To support the healing process, aromatic baths in geranium and rosemary will generally stimulate circulation and the lymphatic system and thereby help to reduce tissue water retention and accelerate detoxification. Acne scars can be treated with a mixture of *wheat germ oil, neroli,* and *lavender* for a combined rejuvenating effect. With this mixture, less visible scars are formed and large, ugly ones are avoided.

Inflammation of the Skin

Inflammations can be caused by injuries, poorly healed wounds, or overexertion, as well as by bacteria and toxic substances that have penetrated the skin. The inflammation may be seen as a plea for attention to the skin.

The appropriate skin oil should contain blue chamomile and a choice of either benzoin, immortelle, and hyssop. Poorly healing wounds should be treated with an anti-inflammatory and wound-healing ointment that has lavender or myrrh added to it. These oils are also used in cool, aromatic baths for dermatitis and superficial inflammations. If the inflammation is accompanied by a painful swelling, make a hot compress with lavender and one of the oils mentioned above.

Itching Skin

What actually causes itching has not yet been completely explained. We only know that some of the many millions of nerve endings act as receptors for itching. We react to itching with scratching, whereby these receptors signal a light pain that temporarily masks the itching. This common symptom occurs particularly after bathing, showering, or swimming.

Many people suffer from itching over the entire body. This condition may be related either to psychological problems (something "driving you crazy"), or to the aggressive substances contained in synthetic soaps, shampoos, shower gels, bath additives, and washing agents, as well as other chemical substances (e.g., chlorine in public swimming pools or tap water). These substances irritate the skin so severly that the acid mantle can be attacked and even completely destroyed when the protective layer of sebum is washed away. The skin and hair suffer especially from the heavily chlorinated water of public swimming pools. After contact with such water, it is very important to thoroughly shower and treat the skin with a lotion. Benzoin, jasmine, Roman chamomile, lavender, peppermint, sandalwood, and cedarwood in aromatic baths, skin oils, and lotions are all helpful for itchy skin, especially Roman chamomile and lavender. Chamomile is a relatively expensive but very effective oil. If only small areas of the skin are frequently plagued by itching, the essential oil may be applied undiluted (as an exception to the general rule).

Eczema

Dry and moist eczema are inflammatory conditions that are often accompanied by itching. Possible causes are oversensitive skin, allergies, psychological troubles, weather influences, and fatigue. In most cases, some degree of psychosomatic irritation is involved. Any subsequent contact with coarse clothing, aggressive washing agents, and chlorinated water encourages further development of eczema.

Moist eczema can be treated with juniper, dry eczema with bergamot, geranium, Roman chamomile, lavender, and melissa. These oils simultaneously calm and strengthen the nerves through the sense of smell. Roman chamomile as well as lavender combat the itching, while bergamot and Roman chamomile inhibit the inflammation. The ideal mixture includes all three of these last-named oils. In cases of intense eczema spread over the entire body, it is best to take an aromatic bath. For minor cases of eczema, make a compress or mix a skin oil to which juniper or rose may be added if crusting or bleeding is present.

Herpes

The swollen lips and the bothersome blisters that regularly occur in the area of the lips, cheeks, and noses of especially susceptible people are manifestations of a virally based skin disease. Herpes is also thought to be promoted by strong solar radiation. People who suffer from herpes should therefore protect their faces from strong ultraviolet radiation. This is the simplest and most certain way of preventing outbreaks.

The healing process for facial herpes can be shortened considerably with pure melissa, dabbed on three times a day. Bergamot, eucalyptus, and tea tree can also be used. Other alternatives are zinc oxide ointment or zinc sulfate. Melissa has been successfully tested for all forms of herpes and can also be used for herpes of the genitals. The latter condition should be treated with a healing ointment made of melissa and rose in a 3:1 proportion, a combination that is also good for shingles.

Psoriasis

Psoriasis is a thickening of the skin caused by a number of factors such as chemical and mechanical irritations, metabolic disturbances, and change of climate, although most cases involve some profound emotional trouble such as deep sorrow or disappointment in response to which the body literally forms a protective barrier against the environment. Highly sensitive people who experience the world as a hostile place are likely to suffer from psoriasis.

The thickening of the skin occurs mostly on the elbows, the knees, the palms of the hands or soles of the feet, around the fingernails, and on the head. It can spread to the connective tissue down to the bones and is externally recognizable as a whitish-yellow elevation. No proven method of treatment guarantees successful healing. Recommended treatments include the use of cedarwood and juniper in the form of skin oil, ultraviolet radiation, and vitamin A (which only fights the symptoms and not the cause). More appropriate would be psychotherapeutic treatment to help bring about a change in the patient's basic attitude toward the world.

Broken Blood Vessels

Due to weakness in the fine blood vessels and through the congestion of blood in the vessel system, red veins may become visible on the surface of the skin as the sign of broken capillary vessels. Their formation is encouraged by spicy foods, alcohol, nicotine, caffeine, pollutants in the air, digestive disturbances, nervous stress, disturbances of the thyroid gland, and vitamin C deficiency.

Neroli, parsley, rose, or Roman chamomile may be added to a skin oil or cream to promote contraction of the blood vessels. This treatment requires much time however, and success is not certain. Facial masks with juniper, camphor, or rosemary may be used to stimulate the blood circulation in the facial skin.

Freckles

Freckles are a whim of nature most often found on light-skinned people. They are not a flaw, but represent rather an entirely natural collection of pigmentation whose function is to protect sensitive skin. If you feel you must treat them, a bleaching effect can be achieved with applications of lemon or onion oil.

Age Spots

The collection of pigmentation in various forms and intensities occurs as a natural development in mature skin. It is promoted by strong doses of ultraviolet radiation and contact with alcohol in the form of perfumes, eau de cologne, commercial cosmetic cleansers rather than soap, and the like. Use vitamin E oil and lemon oil for local treatment, but results will be visible only after long-term regular use. Age spots should be accepted as a natural occurrence in the aging process.

Ultraviolet Radiation, Sun Protection, Sunburn

The sun's natural ultraviolet radiation is important for many bodily functions. Sunlight stimulates proper breathing, circulation, general metabolism, the endocrine gland system, and the formation of vitamin D. This vitamin makes it possible for the body to use calcium from food for strengthening bones, and maintaining the teeth, ligaments, and tendons. Our desire for the sun after long periods of dark, dismal weather or indoor activity is also related to a reaction of the hormonal system, particularly the sexual hormones, which increase our desire for skin contact, tenderness, and sexuality.

Under the effects of ultraviolet radiation, melanocytes in the skin produce the protective pigmentation melanin, which in turn creates the externally visible tanning of the skin. To promote this tanning, cosmetic manufacturers often offer products containing phototoxic or photoallergenic citrus oils such as lemon and bergamot. While these oils do promote tanning under ultraviolet radiation, they should not be used when the sun is very intense since they may then cause dark spots. To tan the skin without strong ultraviolet radiation, add carrot seed oil to creams or oils. Excess ultraviolet radiation causes sunburn, a swelling of the reddened skin that may lead to small or large blisters filled with liquid. In extreme cases, local tissue may die or the DNA (deoxyribonucleinic acid) structure may can be damaged; in the latter case the body can receive false information for the structure of new cells in the process of cell division, which in turn may result in malignant changes in the skin.

As protection for sunbathing, use a mixture of hazelnut oil, sesame oil, wheat germ oil, and vitamin E oil blended with carrot seed and lavender. The oil should be applied about 30 minutes before sunbathing. In case of sunburn, a bath or skin oil containing lavender, peppermint, or lemon will sooth the skin. Even when no burn is present, try a warm bath with lavender, lemon, and almond oil following exposure to sun. Since the hair also dries out under intense solar radiation, it should be given a treatment of almond oil, rosemary, sage, and cedarwood about 15 minutes before washing it.

Varicose Veins

Blue-red, swollen veins are the result of weak circulation and inadequate elasticity in the walls of the veins and membranes, so that the blood cannot easily flow back to the heart. There is congestion and finally inflammation and swelling of the veins. Lack of exercise and the disposition to soft connective tissue encourage their appearance. Varicose veins can be eliminated through compression bandages, electrodessication, or surgery. It is naturally better to prevent them.

If you have weak connective tissue and get little exercise, you need to get your blood vessels, tissue, and muscles "in shape" some other way. Massages, dry brushing, and baths with certain essences can stimulate the circulation and lymph flow. The collected liquids and waste products are then also dissolved, removed, and eliminated. For massage, use cypress, lemon, and calendula oil; do not massage the varicose veins directly but rather the area around them. The legs should be elevated after the massage. Rubbing ointments into the legs or taking an aromatic sitzbath with rosemary, sage, or juniper can also be beneficial. Successful results are obtained with this treatment only when the legs are massaged daily over an extended period of time (for recipe, see page 139).

The following table presents a summary of the healing uses of essential oils for irritations and diseases of the skin and tissue, including functional disturbances not mentioned in the text.

Healing Uses of Essential Oils for Skin Irritations	abscesses	acne	acne wounds	allergy	burns	cellulite	dermatitis	eczema, dry	eczema, moist	freckles	furuncles	herpes	inflamed skin	itching	psoriasis	red, broken vessels	scabs	seborrhea	shingles	sunburn	varicose veins	wounds, healing	wounds, infected
Benzoin	•												•	•									
Bergamot		•						•	•	•									•	•		•	
Cajeput		•																					
Calendula	•	•				•																•	
Camphor																							
Cedarwood		•					•		•				•	•									
Chamomile, blue																						•	•

	abscesses	acne	acne wounds	allergy	burns	cellulite	dermatitis	eczema, dry	eczema, moist	freckles	furuncles	herpes	inflamed skin	itching	psoriasis	red, broken vessels	scabs	seborrhea	shingles	sunburn	varicose veins	wounds, healing	wounds, infected
Chamomile, Roman	•			•							•		•	•	•	•							•
Clary Sage											•		•										
Cypress						•										•		•			•		
Eucalyptus	•												•										
Fennel						•																	
Frankincense																						•	
Garlic	•																•						•
Geranium	•	•			•	•		•						•									
Hyssop							•		•				•									•	
Immortelle					•								•										
Jasmine													•	•									
Juniper		•			•	•		•					•					•			•	•	
Lavender	•	•	•		•			•			•		•	•				•		•		•	
Lemon										•	•			•	•			•		•			
Melissa				•					•			•							•				
Myrrh									•				•				•					•	•
Myrtle		•																					
Neroli			•													•							
Niauoli											•		•										
Onion	•				•					•	•												
Orange						•																	
Oregano						•																	
Parsley							•											•					
Patchouli		•							•				•					•					
Peppermint													•	•									
Rose													•					•					
Rosemary												•										•	•
Sage	•					•														•		•	
Sandalwood													•	•									
Tea Tree		•											•	•									
Thuja											•												
Thyme											•											•	

Cellulite

The unwelcome cellulite that forms on the thighs, hips, and buttocks of women is flabby, spongy tissue, the result of lymph congestion, decreased elimination of waste products and toxins, water retention in the connective tissue, and an increase in fatty tissue production. Cellulite is often associated with dull pain, and feelings of heaviness and tension, as well as sensitivity to pain when pressed or pushed. It is not an illness in the strict sense.

Treatment of cellulite aims to remove water, reduce fat, and activate the functions of the connective tissue and circulation. Taking vitamin E, inositol-phosphatide, and choline regulates the cellular water equilibrium and counteracts fatty degeneration. It is also useful to jog and do leg or hip exercises on a regular basis. The natural cosmetic approach is to massage the affected body parts daily and have an aromatic bath twice a week with oils that stimulate the metabolism and circulation, removing excessive liquids. Fennel, juniper, and cypress remove these excessive liquids; geranium, parsley, rosemary, orange, oregano, and sage tone and stimulate circulation and metabolism (for recipes, see pages 136–137).

Essential Oils for Skin Care

Hands and Nails

Hands are probably the most frequently used and versatile "tool" of the body. That is why the palms are covered with a thick horny layer of epithelium to protect them from injuries and penetrating germs, acids, lyes, and dirt. Yet the body's own protection is sometimes inadequate and needs to be supported with natural products. For cleansing, use lemon, for skin care Roman chamomile, lavender, and rose. Myrrh is excellent for brittle, chapped, or injured skin.

The nails protect the hands and feet by providing a first point of sensory contact with the environment, and also extend their capability to grasp. Like the hair, they contain a tough protein called keratin and grow about 0.02 inches a week (more quickly in the summer than in the winter). Healthy nails are elastic, have a dull shine, and are slightly curved. White moons and a rosy coloring are signs of good blood circulation and optimal metabolism. In contrast, tears, ridges, white spots, blue-red coloring, and the like can indicate high blood pressure, presence of toxic substances, inadequate intestinal function, and a lack of calcium. Breakage-prone nails can be strengthened by periodical soaking in lemon or onion oil. Smoothness, shine, and healthy growth are attained with lavender, sandalwood, or cypress. All treatments use vegetable oils mixed with a few drops of essential oils (recipes for the care and cleansing of hands and for nail care are on pages 126–129).

Feet

Whatever applies to the hands also applies to the feet. Surely no other part of the body is as overburdened as the feet. Few people take care of their feet yet we expect them always to function: perhaps our negligence is related to the fact that modern Western society puts more emphasis on the role of the head.

One recommendation is to have regular and thorough massages with special skin oils (see "Shiatsu Massage for Beauty," page 147). Foot baths are a true treat, and particularly provide relief for people who have to walk or stand a good portion of the time. Such baths also counteract unpleasant foot odor, which can be remedied above all with pine and cypress. Lavender and sage can also be used. For tired, aching feet, use lavender, clary sage, peppermint, juniper, or rosemary. In the case of severe foot odor and pain, a special cream for the feet can be prepared from these oils.

Few people are aware that when the feet are in healthy condition, the skin benefits as well. The feet contain reflex zones for every organ of the body. By specifically treating certain areas of the feet, you can influence the entire body. Make sure that the outermost skin layer does not become too thick and chapped. Rough skin can be removed by rubbing it with a pumice stone or a

special skin file, which then improves the circulation and the
metabolism. In addition, you will also have better "contact" with
the floor.

Try the following five-minute foot exercise to increase the
circulation and relax the muscles: circle with the left foot and then
the right foot in both directions; contract and then relax the toes;
move your feet back and forth, as far as they will go. Repeat ten
times. (For treatment of corns, blisters, athlete's foot, and warts, see
pages 135–139.)

Mouth and Teeth

The flora of the mouth contain bacteria that actually initiate the
digestive process, while the saliva keeps the mouth moist in order
to let the bacteria grow. At the smell of food, we secrete saliva
composed in response to the specific type of smell. However, other
bacteria having nothing to do with the digestive process can form
in the mouth through inflammation of the gums, abscesses, or
infections of the pharynx. These not only harm the mouth bacteria, but also create a bad taste in the mouth and bad breath. Other
causes for bad breath are digestive disturbances and stomach diseases, but rarely food remnants between the teeth.

Cleaning the teeth should actually just have the purpose of
removing food remnants and film from the teeth, as well as massaging the gums. The whiteners, preservatives, and foaming agents
contained in most tooth-care products attack the gums and mouth
flora, killing the bacteria that promote digestion. Natural tooth-care
products contain only abrasives (such as salt, chalk, siliceous earth),
binding agents (such as glycerine), and herbal extracts or essential
oils that strengthen the gums by stimulating circulation, freshen the
breath, and have a slightly antiseptic effect.

For bad breath, try a mouthwash containing bergamot, eucalyptus, fennel, myrrh, peppermint, or thyme. For inflammations of the
mouth or pharynx, use the antiseptic oils bergamot and lavender in
mouthwash form. Fennel, sage, and thyme are particularly suited
for taking care of the gums. (For mouthwash recipes, see page 130.)

Recipes for Skin Care

In choosing these recipes, I have selected those that are the simplest
to make. My own experience with facial and body oils has shown
me that jojoba oil blended with essential oils is simple to make and
very efficient for skin care, moisturizing, and rejuvenating. Such
mixtures work just as well as oil-based creams and are suitable for
all types of skin. Jojoba oil is relatively expensive, but goes the
furthest in taking care of your skin. For those who prefer to make
creams, recipes are given as well. *The amounts of essential oils in the
recipes are always given in drops*: thus "10 bergamot" means 10 drops
of bergamot oil.

In making creams or lotions, you will occasionally notice that the
contents separate; this is especially likely to occur at room temperature. Simply stir the cream briefly with a clean object and use it as
soon as possible. Shake all lotions before using! Natural emulsifiers
are not as perfect as their chemical substitutes.

When preparing cosmetics, feel free to make larger amounts.
These can be stored in a cool place, while only the amount needed
for immediate use should be kept in the bathroom. If a cream or
lotion does not become as stiff as you are accustomed to in store
products, don't question your abilities as a cosmetic maker. The
ingredients will still work. Also check the recipes for notes on how
to change the consistency of various products.

One note about "moisturizing": you can only moisturize the
surface of the skin, but the subcutis or the tissue will not become
any more moist than it already is. Moisturizing creams or lotions
are applied to help avoid the loss of moisture. It is the fat content
which fulfills this function. In other words, any cream or oil based
on some fat content will automatically help to regulate the moisture of the skin.

It is essential in planning skin treatment to pay attention to the
inner clock that regulates all body functions. Our skin cells are
naturally more burdened during the day, when the body must be in
"full swing." In the evening, when the body gradually calms down,

and especially at night when we sleep, the cells can best recover and renew themselves. This is why nutritive and regenerative creams, skin oils, and healing oils should be applied in the evening.

Skin Cleansing

When cleansing the skin, pay particular attention to the skin type involved (see page 75). If water and soap, are used, choose a soap that is free of alkalines and nonirritating to the skin. The best types are soft soap made of coconut fat and soda soap made from cattle sebum, better known as liquid soap. Buy a "pure" soap or "natural soap." Synthetic, perfumed soaps, even the most expensive products, do not wash any better. Deodorant soaps or synthetic soaps are not ideal, and alcohol should fundamentally be avoided. Be aware that if the hands are employed directly in cleansing, they can actually serve to carry dirt into the pores in the process. For this reason tissues or cotton balls are recommended for applying and removing excess cleansing cream or lotion.

Flower waters (lavender, rose, and orange blossom) and witch hazel work very well for facial cleansing, since they are antiseptic, anti-inflammatory, soothing, cooling, and toning.

Cleansing Oil

This oil is good to use for gentle cleansing of the facial skin.

Ingredients:

> 2 oz. almond oil or jojoba oil
> 15–20 drops of essential oil, alone or in combination: peppermint, basil, juniper, lemon, and tea tree for blemished skin

Procedure:

Put all ingredients in an amber-colored bottle and shake well. For cleansing, put some of the oil on the face and remove with a cotton ball.

Cleansing Lotion

Ingredients:

> 4 oz. witch hazel solution or flower water
> 20 drops essential oil

Procedure:

Place all ingredients into a bottle and shake well. For very oily skin, use 10 drops of camphor, 5 drops of thyme, and 5 drops of peppermint. For normal, dry, or mixed skin, use a mixture of juniper, basil, peppermint, and/or lemon.

The flower waters of lavender, orange blossom, and rose can be made into very pleasant-scented facial lotions that not only cleanse but also have a toning and astringent effect. You can give free rein to your fantasy and creativity, making wonderfully fragrant mixtures with flower waters and essential oils. The result is an eau de toilette that doubles as a skin cleanser and toner. Apply the cleansing lotion to your face and neck with a cotton ball, then rub it off with gentle motions.

Toning Cleansing Lotion

This cleansing lotion can be especially effective for blemished and oily skin.

Ingredients:

> 15 oz. distilled or boiled water or flower water
> ½ oz. apple cider vinegar
> 20 peppermint
> 20 juniper
> Yield: 16 oz.

Procedure:

Pour the mixture into a bottle and shake well, and a portion can be conveniently kept in a small bottle with a spray top. The rest can be stored in the refrigerator.

Apply this cleansing lotion with a cotton ball and rub the face and neck with gentle motions. Or spray the face with a spray bottle and after a few minutes blot dry with a cotton ball. The more apple cider vinegar you use, the more its scent will dominate the mixture. It will then also have more of a toning effect, and the skin will feel smooth and fresh afterward. For severely blemished skin, use tea tree or lemon instead of peppermint. Gentle cleansing with vinegar and essential oils aims at stimulating the skin functions. The lotion has a stronger effect when prepared with lemon, so this mixture is not suitable for sensitive skin.

To cleanse the body, use a mild, natural soap. Many types of pure and natural soaps are now available—olive soaps, lavender soaps, almond soaps, and so on—or you can buy a non-irriting soft soap and perfume it yourself. In the section "Recipes for Aromatic Baths," you will find recipes for cleansing baths (see page 130).

Liquid Soaps

This very simple recipe calls for 1 cup of liquid soap as a base. Use either white soft soap or a nonirritating liquid soap, or melt a piece of natural soap. Add ½ cup of water and 5 drops of essential oils. I recommend a refreshing fragrance such as lemon, lemongrass, orange, peppermint, or lavender. Shake the solution thoroughly in a bottle with a spray top.

For dry skin and hard water, add 1 to 2 tablespoons of of almond oil to the mixture so that the soap will replace the fat taken from the skin. This prevents tight, dry skin and itching. These liquid soaps can be used to wash the entire body.

Shower and Washing Gel

This shower gel is a bit more complicated to make than the liquid soap.

Ingredients:

  85 g glycerine
  15 g pectin
  85 g liquid soap

2 tbsp. vegetable oil (optional)
2 g borax (optional)
10 drops essential oils
Yield: about 7 oz.

Procedure:

Heat the glycerine slowly in a heatproof bowl. Slowly sprinkle in the pectin powder while stirring rapidly. Be sure there are no lumps. When the mass is homogeneous, add the vegetable oil, the liquid soap, and the essential oils while continuing to stir. Pour the mass into a bottle with a spray or pump top. If the gel becomes too firm, it can be diluted later by gradually stirring in water.

To make a larger batch, simply double the recipe. Choose your favorite scent for this shower gel: try a flowery fragrance such as lavender, rose, neroli, or jasmine; a refreshing scent such such as lemon, citronella, lemongrass, orange, petitgrain, or peppermint; or a woody fragrance such as sandalwood, cedarwood, cypress, rosewood, or oak moss.

Facial Steam Baths

The steam bath is an old and proven method for cleansing the skin. The damp warmth stimulates prespiration and thus flushes out dirt, toxic substances, and skin scales. Steam baths guarantee deep pore cleansing, stimulate circulation, and moisturize the skin, while the scent of the essential oils they contain is refreshing.

For the steam bath, use oils that are appropriate for your skin type or a general cleansing oil such as peppermint, juniper, or lemon. For dry and sensitive skin, don't make the steam bath too hot and limit the time to 5 minutes at most. You can apply steam to normal skin for 7 minutes and to oily skin for up to 10 minutes. After a steam bath the skin will be soft, with good blood circulation, and very receptive to further care in the form of a light cream, toner, oil, or a facial pack. Use only small amounts so that the skin can breathe.

The start of winter is a good time for a steam bath containing a stimulating oil such as rosemary or sage. Simply boil 1 to 2 pints of water. Place the partially cooled water into a bowl, add about 10 drops of essential oils, bend over the bowl, and cover your head and the bowl with a towel so that no steam escapes. Here are three recipes for stimulation and one for cleansing:

Steam Bath for Normal Skin

> 4 lavender
> 4 geranium
> 4 bergamot

Steam Bath for Oily Skin and Acne

> 6 juniper
> 4 lemon
> 4 cypress

Steam Bath for Mature Skin and Wrinkles

> 6 neroli
> 4 lavender

Cleansing Steam Bath

> 4 peppermint
> 2 camphor
> 4 juniper

Facial Compresses

Facial compresses have the same effect as steam baths. They stimulate the skin, moisten it, and swell the cornified layer of the epithelium; the essential oils are then more quickly absorbed by the skin. The face should be cleansed before applying the compresses. Following this treatment, the skin is soft, smooth, and receptive to further care.

Heat about 2 pints of water to the boiling point and allow it to cool briefly. Add 3 to 4 drops of essential oils, stir briefly. Now dip a small terry towel into the water, wring it out lightly (so that it no longer drips), and put it on your face. The pot may be left on the stove over a small flame. When the compress cools off, dip the towel in again.

If the skin is very dry, mature, or sensitive, use only lukewarm compresses. Following this treatment you can massage the face, gently press any blackheads, treat the skin with a mild facial lotion, or apply a light cream or oil but no makeup. The skin should be given the opportunity to breathe. Here are some suggestions for mixing essential oils:

For Normal Skin

> 2 lavender
> 2 bergamot

For Dry Skin

> 1 rose
> 2 Roman chamomile
> 1 neroli
> (lukewarm)

For Oily Skin

> 1 rose
> 2 geranium
> 1 sandalwood

For Inflamed, Sensitive Skin

> 2 blue chamomile
> 1 myrrh
> 1 rose

For Mature Skin and Wrinkles

> 2 frankincense
> 2 neroli

or
2 myrrh

For Blemished Skin and Acne

2 juniper
2 lavender
or
1 lemon
3 bergamot
or
4 tea tree

Facial Oils

Facial oils are simple to make and have the same effects as creams. Moreover, they last longer and are absorbed well and quickly by the skin. The combination of a high-quality vegetable oil and essential oils guarantees optimal skin care and healing effects. The vegetable oil serves as a solvent for essential oils, helping them to penetrate quickly and without residue. At the same time, the vegetable oil provides the skin with nutrients (vitamins, essential fatty acids, etc.) and regulates its moisture balance.

I recommend jojoba oil for its superior effect and high yield. Sweet almond oil should also be mentioned here as an excellent — and considerably less expensive—choice. The advantage of jojoba oil, aside from its unsurpassed effect on hair and skin, is that it is absorbed quickly by the skin and leaves no residue. Only a light, silky shine remains. Almond oil takes longer to be absorbed and leaves an oily film on certain types of skin after the recommended 15 minutes of time it needs to work. The extra oil should be removed with a cotton ball.

A very good skin care formula is a blend of jojoba oil and 10% wheat germ oil with vitamin E. (As a matter of principle, I always add some vitamin E oil to facial oils.) The following recipes are based upon 2 ounces of vegetable oil and about 20 drops of essential oils, which are placed in an amber-colored bottle and shaken well. To make a larger quantity, simply double the recipe.

These blends do not have to be stored in a cool place since they rarely become rancid.

For Normal Skin

> 15 lavender
> 8 geranium
> 4 rose
> *or*
> 15 cedarwood
> 10 rosewood
> *or*
> 10 rose
> 5 rosewood
> 5 geranium

For Dry Skin

> 10 sandalwood
> 7 geranium
> 5 ylang-ylang
> 3 rosewood
> *or*
> 10 rose
> 5 jasmine
> 5 geranium
> *or*
> 10 cedarwood
> 10 sandalwood
> 5 rosewood
> 10% wheat germ oil

For Oily Skin

> 15 lemon
> 10 cypress
> *or*

10 lavender
10 camphor
or
10 bergamot
10 orange
5 geranium

For Inflamed Skin

10 blue or Roman chamomile
10 lavender
or
10 sandalwood
5 blue or Roman chamomile
5 cedarwood
or
15 patchouli
5 myrrh
1 clove

For Mature Skin

15 lavender
5 frankincense
5 neroli
or
20 carrot seed
5 myrrh
or
10 patchouli
10 frankincense

For Wrinkles

15 fennel
5 lavender
5 rose

or
15 frankincense
5 cypress
10% wheat germ oil or vitamin E oil

For Acne, Blemished Skin

15 bergamot
10 juniper
5 cypress
 or
15 tea tree
10 lavender
 or
15 patchouli
5 Roman chamomile
5 cedarwood

For Irritated, Sensitive Skin

15 Roman chamomile
5 carrot seed
5 bergamot
 or
15 orange
5 neroli
5 lavender

All-Purpose Oil for Facial Cleansing and Body Care

This oil can be used as a skin oil, moisturizer, massage oil, and bath oil. It is made of superior skin care oils and nutrient oils such as aloe vera, with its anti-inflammatory and healing substances. It is suitable for every skin type, but can be particularly recommended for irritated, dry, sore, and inflamed skin.

Ingredients:

> 75 g jojoba oil
> 15 g wheat germ oil
> 15 g almond oil
> 15 g avocado oil
> 15 g sunflower oil
> 15 g vitamin E oil
> 60 g aloe vera
> 30 g glycerine
> Yield: about 9 oz.

Procedure:

Combine oils and warm to 160°F. At the same time, heat the glycerine and aloe vera to 160°F. Take both mixtures from the water bath and add the oil mixture to the aloe vera–glycerine while rapidly stirring. Keep stirring until the mixture cools down to about 100°F. If the water and oil separate later, shake the bottle vigorously before use.

This all-purpose oil can be made completely of jojoba oil and wheat germ oil. Small amounts can be taken as needed from this basic blend and used to create various skin care products by adding essential oils. For example, to every 2 ounces of a cleansing, skin care, or massage oil add about 20 drops of essential oils. For an aromatic bath, add 2 to 3 tablespoons of the oil and a few drops of essential oils to the bath water; or a ready-made bath mixture can be prepared by blending 4 ounces of the all-purpose oil with about 60 drops of essential oils. For a healing oil (e.g., for inflamed skin or severe acne), prepare a 3% solution—that is, about 60 drops of essential oils to 2 ounces of basic oil.

Facial Lotion and Body Lotion

This basic recipe for four ounces of facial lotion can be individualized by adding essential oils; a body lotion can be made simply by increasing the recipe volume. More water can be added if a thinner facial lotion is desired. It is very moisturizing.

Ingredients:

>   40 g avocado or jojoba oil
>   30 g rosewater or another flower water
>   30 g lanolin
>   20—30 drops essential oils
>   Yield: about 4 oz.

Procedure:

Heat lanolin in a double boiler until a thin liquid is obtained. Add the vegetable oil and stir slowly over medium heat. At the same time, heat rosewater to the same temperature. Then slowly add the rosewater to the other mixture while under rapid continual stirring. Before it cools completely, add the essential oils and mix again briefly. Pour into a bottle and store in a cool place. Choose essential oils that correspond to your skin type.

Facial Care with Creams

The difficulty in making creams from water and oil is how to bind them into a homogeneous mass—a problem manufactures of synthetic cosmetics resolve by using chemical emulsifiers. Since our recipes use only natural substances, the key lies rather in careful attention to precision of temperature (whenever given) and even mixing (medium speed for an electric mixer). Once the creams have been refrigerated for a time, drops of water may appear on the surface—a sign that the essential oils have replaced some of the water content. These can be blotted with a cotton swab or simply allowed to evaporate.

Facial Creams Containing Sweet Cream

Sweet cream is actually the best basic substance for making facial creams. In fact, cream was the predecessor of our current ready-made creams (hence the name), and it contains much nutrition for the skin: vitamins, minerals, fats, and protein. Use only fresh, heavy sweet cream. This cream only lasts a few days and should therefore be made in small amounts. It is simple to prepare: mix about 2 ounces with 5 to 10 drops of essential oils (chosen by skin type), place the cream in a small jar and refrigerate. Note that real cream can also be used on oily skin.

For sensitive skin, add about 5 drops jasmine or rose; for normal skin, 10 drops lavender; for blemished skin, 5 drops camphor or 10 of tea tree; use 10 drops bergamot for oily skin; 10 drops frankincense or patchouli for mature skin; and 10 drops sandalwood or geranium for dry skin.

Skin Care and Cleansing Creams

One of the oldest recipes handed down to us (150 A.D.) is a cream devised by the famous physician Claudius Galenus. This recipe, still the basis of cleansing creams today, is called cold cream because of its cooling effect. It is surprisingly easy to make, and the ingredients are not expensive (which may lead one to wonder why commercially produced creams cost so much).

Ingredients:

50 g almond oil
25 g beeswax
about 15–20 g distilled water or flower water
2 g borax
20–30 drops of essential oils
Yield: about 4 oz.

Procedure:

Melt the wax and oil in a double boiler. Stir the mixture and remove from heat. Now gradually add the water and borax (dissoved in a small amount of water beforehand), stirring rapidly, until the cream reaches the desired consistency. The amount of water can be varied to obtain a thinner or thicker cream, as desired.

Finally, add a favorite fragrance from among the classic cleansing oils: basil, juniper, peppermint, lemon, and niauoli. After application remove the cleansing cream with cotton balls and wash the face thoroughly with warm water.

The skin care cream can be refined further by using jojoba oil instead of almond oil and by the addition of honey to smooth, soothe, and nourish the skin. Add 2 tablespoons of honey to the oil solution and use correspondingly less water. I have discovered that this refined cream, very thinly applied, is also suitable for skin care, and particularly good for hot days.

Jojoba Cleansing Cream

The following basic recipe can be altered by substituting oils with a favorite scent or those corresponding to a particular skin type. It is also suitable for use as a treatment cream for very dry skin. (Use the appropriate oils for dry skin.)

Ingredients:

> 80 g jojoba oil
> 8 g beeswax
> 20 g cocoa butter
> 20 drops essential oils: pepper, juniper, basil, lemon
> (mix as desired)
> Yield: about 4 oz.

Procedure:

Melt the beeswax in a double boiler. Add the oil and cocoa butter and mix well. Now remove from the heat and continue to stir slowly until the mass cools down somewhat. Add essential oils and stir again. Pour into a container and store in a cool place. After application, remove the cream with a cotton ball and rinse the face with plenty of warm water. Although the above cleansing cream is suitable for all skin types, I recommend the following cleansing lotion for oily skin.

Witch Hazel Cleansing Cream for Blemished Skin

This cream has a healing, toning, anti-inflammatory, and astringent effect.

Ingredients:

> 40 g jojoba oil
> 40 g witch hazel solution
> 10 g beeswax
> 1 tsp. vitamin E oil
> 1 g borax
> 10 tea tree
> 10 juniper or basil
> Yield: about 4 oz.

Procedure:

Heat beeswax and oils to 160°F in the top of a double boiler, stirring constantly. At the same time, mix borax and witch hazel solution and warm to 160°F (also in a double boiler). Remove both mixtures from the heat and slowly add the oil blend to the water mixture while stirring rapidly.

When the cream has cooled down to about 110°F, add the essential oils and stir again. Fill into containers (this amount is best divided into two batches) and store in a cool place. Apply the cream sparingly. After a few minutes wipe it away with a cotton ball. Finish by rinsing with warm water.

Moisturizing Cream

A moisturizer should be applied after every washing, shower, or bath, since the oil film on the skin is washed away in the process. The following creams protect against moisture loss, stabilizes the acid mantle, and keeps dirt from clogging the pores.

Witch Hazel Moisturizer

This cream is good for mature, tired, clogged, blemished, and inflamed skin. Its effect is astringent, toning, protective, and healing.

Ingredients:

> 30 g almond oil
> 3 g lanolin

25 g beeswax
1 tbsp. vitamin E oil
180 g witch hazel solution
5 g glycerine
2 g borax
40–50 drops of essential oils
Yield: about 10 oz.

Procedure:

Mix witch hazel solution, glycerine, and borax. Heat to 175°F in a double boiler. Heat almond oil, lanolin, beeswax, and vitamin E oil in a second double boiler to 175°F and stir. Remove both mixtures from the heat and slowly pour the water mixture into the oil mixture while stirring constantly. Keep stirring until the cream has cooled to about 100°F. Add the essential oils (chosen by skin type or preferred fragrance), stir again briefly, fill into a container, and refrigerate.

Jojoba–Aloe Vera Moisturizer

Jojoba–aloe vera moisturizer is absorbed very quickly. Anti-inflammatory, healing, and toning, this skin care cream leaves the skin silky and soft. It is suitable for every skin type and even without the addition or essential oils has a pleasant cocoa butter scent. It rarely turns rancid.

Ingredients:

25 g jojoba oil
10 g beeswax
10 g cocoa butter
1 tbsp. vitamin E oil
50 g aloe vera
10 g glycerine
20—30 drops essential oils
Yield: about 4 oz.

Procedure:

Heat jojoba oil, beeswax, cocoa butter, and vitamin E oil to 160°F in a double boiler and mix. Mix aloe vera and glycerine in a second double boiler and heat to 160°F. Then take the mixtures from the stove and add the oil mixture dropwise to the aloe vera–glycerine mixture while constantly stirring. Keep stirring until the cream has cooled down to about 80°F, then add the essential oils. Stir again briefly, fill into a container, and refrigerate.

Skin Care Creams

Day Cream

The following basic recipe can be personalized with a favorite fragrance or turned into a multipurpose cream by selecting oils according to skin type (see page 75) or skin problem (see page 82). Or let your nose decide—it knows best what is good for you. A rose cream is not merely a skin care cream but can actually open the heart with its scent; melissa cream, is especially refreshing and invigorating in the morning.

Ingredients:

> 40 g jojoba oil
> 40 g witch hazel solution, flower water, or aloe vera
> 15 g lanolin
> 6 g beeswax
> 20–30 drops essential oils
> Yield: about 4 oz.

Procedure:

Heat beeswax, lanolin, and jojoba oil in a double boiler until everything has melted. Stir briefly. Remove from the heat and blend in a mixer or blender on lowest speed. Add the witch hazel solution, flower water, or aloe vera by drops. Stir until the mixture is almost cold and solidified. Add the essential oils, stir again, place in a container, and refrigerate.

I recommend the following combinations of waters and essential oils: for normal skin, rose water with geranium and rose or bergamot and lavender with witch hazel solution; for oily skin, witch hazel solution with camphor, juniper, or rosemary; for blemished skin and acne, aloe vera, camphor, tea tree, or lavender; for mature skin, rose water with cypress, frankincense, or rose; for dry skin, aloe vera with ylang-ylang, sandalwood, or jasmine; for mature skin and wrinkles, orange blossom water with neroli, frankincense, myrrh, or lavender; for inflamed and blemished skin, witch hazel.

Carrot Seed Nutritive Cream

This cream is moisturizing, toning, soothing, and protective.

Ingredients:

>   40 g almond oil or jojoba oil
>   40 g rose water
>   15 g lanolin
>   5 g beeswax
>   20—25 drops carrot seed
>   Yield: about 4 oz.

Procedure:

Made like the rejuvenation cream below (see page 115).

Rose Cream

A pure rose cream is made like the carrot seed nutritive cream (see above), using 20 drops of rose oil. This cream is particularly good for dry and sensitive skin.

Rejuvenation Cream

This moisturizing and rejuvenating cream is best applied in the evening before going to sleep, since the skin absorbs the active ingredients best at that time.

Ingredients:

>   40 g rose water
>   20 g jojoba oil
>   10 g wheat germ oil
>   10 g lanolin

5 g cocoa butter
5 g beeswax
1 tbsp. honey
20–30 drops essential oils
Yield: about 4 oz.

Procedure:

Melt beeswax, cocoa butter, and lanolin in a double boiler until a clear liquid forms. Add the jojoba oil and wheat germ oil and slowly stir when the temperature reaches 140°F. At the same time, heat the rose water in a second double boiler to 140°F. Remove both mixtures from the heat and slowly add the rose water to the oil mixture while constantly stirring, until the mass is skin temperature. Add honey and essential oils, stir again briefly, place into container and refrigerate. Frankincense, patchouli, rose, neroli, and lavender are the oils to use for rejuvenation. Of course, 60–80 drops of any essential oils can be added to create a healing cream.

Rejuvenation Aloe Vera Night Cream

This cream combines the oils of the rejuvenation cream with aloe vera, which has an anti-inflammatory, healing effect. It is a night cream for every type of skin, but can be particularly recommended for irritated, sensitive skin.

Ingredients:

20 g almond oil
20 g cocoa butter
1 tbsp. vitamin E oil
10 g jojoba oil
4 g beeswax
130 g aloe vera
10 g glycerine
40–45 drops essential oils
(see rejuvenation cream, page 114)
Yield: about 7 oz.

Procedure:

Heat cocoa butter, oils, and wax to 175°F while stirring constantly. At the same time, warm glycerine and aloe vera in another pot to the same temperature while constantly stirring. Take both mixtures from the stove. Now slowly stir the water mixture into the oil mixture and continue to stir until it has cooled down to 100°F. Add the essential oils, stir again, fill into container (or several small containers), and refrigerate.

Jojoba Skin Protection Cream

The skin easily becomes dry with changing weather conditions and during travel. Under such circumstances it requires additional moisture in the form of fat. The following skin protection cream provides a protective and moisture-regulating film. The best time to apply a skin protection cream is before you go to bed. Lips can be treated with pure lanolin, wheat germ oil, or cocoa butter.

Ingredients:

> 60 g jojoba oil
> 15 g beeswax
> 1–2 tsp. honey
> 20 carrot seed
> Yield: about 2 ½ oz.

Procedure:

Heat the beeswax and jojoba oil until it becomes a clear mass. Pour into a bowl and mix well until it has cooled to skin temperature. Add the carrot seed oil and honey, stir again, and fill into a container. The mass becomes creamy after a short time.

Facial Lotion

Here is a facial lotion to refresh and stimulate the skin functions. It should be applied after cleansing and can also be used as a substitute for oil when the skin is very greasy. I recommend a mixture of 8 ounces of distilled or pure water and 25 drops of essential oil; instead of distilled water, witch hazel solution may be used, in which case the lotion will have an astringent effect. For dry skin, add vegetable oil to this mixture (to 5–10% of the total) and shake well before using. Equal parts of witch hazel solution and aloe vera make a toning, astringent, and healing mixture for inflamed skin.

Here are some suggestions for essential oils that work well in a facial lotion: for dry and normal skin, 15 lavender, 10 geranium, 5 bergamot or jasmine; for oily skin, 15 bergamot and 10 lavender; for sensitive skin, 15 Roman chamomile and 5 jasmine; for acne and blemished skin, 15 juniper and 10 tea tree; and for mature skin, 10 frankincense, 10 myrrh, and 5 patchouli.

Flower Water

Facial lotions can also be made with flower water and honey. Here is a mild and wonderfully fragrant facial lotion for every skin type: its effect is soothing, astringent, and anti-inflammatory. The effect of the added honey is nutritive, smoothing, and slightly antiseptic.

Ingredients:

> 4 oz. orange blossom water
> 2 tsp. honey
> 2 bergamot
> Yield: about 4 oz.

Procedure:

Heat the flower water, dissolve the honey in it, fill it into a bottle, add the essential oil, and shake the contents well. This recipe can be combined with lavender water, rose water, orange blossom water, and the essential oil fragrances that best suit your type.

Lavender water harmonizes with lemon, orange, clary sage, and rosemary; rose water harmonizes with bergamot, geranium, jasmine, patchouli, rosewood, and sandalwood; orange blossom water harmonizes with bergamot, geranium, lavender, neroli, clary sage, and petitgrain.

Aftershave Lotion

After shaving, the facial skin needs a soothing, astringent, and anti-inflammatory lotion. The best base is witch hazel solution.

Ingredients:

> 4 oz. witch hazel solution
> 10–20 ml pure grain alcohol (optional;
>   never use for dry skin)
> 15–20 drops essential oils
> Yield: about 4 oz.

Procedure:

Put all of the ingredients into a bottle and shake well. Men usually prefer essential oils with woody scents such as sandalwood, oak moss, and cedarwood. I always add two drops of the antiseptic clove oil or cinnamon to my aftershave lotion.

Made with jojoba oil, the lotion is also anti-inflammatory, moisturizing, and beneficial to the skin. I prefer this lotion because it is like a facial lotion and an aftershave cream in one.

For a total yield of 3 ounces, try one of the following mixtures: 1 clove, 15 cedarwood, and 5 bergamot; 1 clove, 15 sandalwood, and 5 frankincense; 1 clove, 5 sandalwood, 10 cedarwood, 5 ylang-ylang; or try 1 cinnamon and 1 clove instead of just 1 clove.

Masks

Masks should cleanse and tauten the skin, promote circulation, and generally invigorate. Their effect is very intense if you use Fuller's earth or clay; hence a gel mask is preferable for sensitive skin.

Masks are particularly beneficial for oily and blemished skin. Avoid applying to the area around the eyes, since the skin here is too thin and would be strained and dried out by a mask. Leave the mask on the facial skin for about 15 minutes, or until completely dry. Then remoisten thoroughly and carefully wash it off, using a damp wash-cloth and rinsing generously with much warm water afterward.

Finally, a refreshing facial water may be applied, but *no* cream or oil, so that the skin can breathe. Masks are best applied in the evening, since the skin is particularly receptive to nutrients at that time. Use this time to relax (try letting the mask work while soaking in the tub, for example).

The most important ingredient of the classic mask is clay. It works like a magnet, pulling dirt and toxic substances out of the skin. Clay contains valuable minerals such as iron, magnesium, zinc, potassium, calcium, and silica acid. Any of the following ingredients may be added to it:

Almond oil: regulates skin moisture, for very dry skin

Aloe vera: healing, beneficial to skin, rejuvenating for all skin types

Avocado: nutritive, for dry, normal, sensitive, and mature skin

Egg white: nutritive, for sensitive skin

Egg yolk: for dry skin

Flower water: astringent, toning, soothing for irritated skin, for all skin types

Glycerine: regulates skin moisture, oily skin

Honey: regulates skin moisture, nutritive, smoothing, removes dirt, for all skin types, particularly blemished, dry, or sensitive skin

Jojoba oil: regulates skin moisture, healing, for all skin types, for acne

Lemon: refreshing, reduces fat, cleanses, for tired skin

Wheat germ oil: for mature skin, wrinkles, dry skin

Witch hazel solution: astringent, soothes irritated skin, for all skin types

Yogurt: nutritive, regulates skin moisture, for acne, sensitive, oily, or pale skin

Following guidelines for the use of essential oils to promote skin care and healing effects in the particular skin type being treated, add 4 drops of oil: for example, use lavender, bergamot, rose, and jasmine for normal skin; thyme, camphor, juniper, tea tree, lemon, and bergamot for acne; lavender, Roman chamomile, and rose for sensitive skin or for red, broken veins; carrot seed, rose, and sandalwood for dry skin; frankincense, patchouli, and cypress for mature skin; rosemary, camphor, eucalyptus, juniper, and frankincense for oily skin and (oily) seborrhea.

Procedure:

Prepare a mask by putting 2 to 3 tablespoons of clay in a small bowl. Then add the fruit pulp, yogurt, honey, essential oils and liquids to make a paste that can be applied to the skin. If the paste is too thin, gradually add more clay. Here are the recipes:

For Normal, Dry, and Sensitive Skin

> 2 tbsp. clay
> 1 tsp. honey or avocado oil
> 2 tsp. water or jojoba oil or aloe vera
> 2 lavender
> 2 bergamot

For Acne, Blemished Skin

> 2 tbsp. clay
> 1 tsp. yogurt
> 2 tsp. jojoba oil or water
> 2 juniper
> 2 bergamot

For Mature Skin

> 2 tbsp. clay
> 1 tbsp. honey
> 2 tsp. water
> 2 frankincense
> 2 neroli

For Oily Skin

> 2 tbsp. clay
> 1 tsp. lemon (fruit pulp)
> 1 tsp. honey
> 1 tsp. water
> 2 juniper
> 2 camphor

Packs

Packs are soft, porous masks that do not dry on the skin. They cleanse the pores, stimulate circulation, and tauten the skin. A pack can cover the entire face. Instead of clay, use one of the nutritive creams or aloe vera, glycerine, or jojoba oil. You can leave the pack on the cleansed facial skin for half an hour. Wash it off and rinse with lukewarm water afterward.

Ingredients:

> 2 tbsp. nutritive cream
> 1 tsp. honey or yogurt or fruit pulp
> 1 tsp. aloe vera or jojoba oil or water
> 4 drops essential oils

Procedure:

Follow the recipe for masks (page 120); the choice of essential oils is also the same.

Peeling

Peeling is recommended on a regular basis for acne or blemished skin with poor circulation. The upper skin layer with its dead scales is gently rubbed off. The pores become free, pimples open, and sebum is released. After peeling, the skin is stimulated, soft, and smooth. It is best to thoroughly cleanse the skin, possibly even with a steam bath, before peeling.

The ingredients for peeling are the following: almond bran with yogurt, finely grated almonds with honey or cream, blue clay, yeast; the best liquids to use are lavender water and 4 to 6 drops of tea tree or 3 drops of camphor.

Procedure:

Mix a paste (see recipe for masks on page 120) and cover the entire face with the exception of the throat, lips, and area around the eyes. After 10 minutes, when the mask has dried completely, wash it away with a moistened sponge or with gentle circling motions of the hand. A facial toner or facial oil may be applied afterward.

Now some recipes for body care:

Body Oils and Lotions

The same general directions apply for making body oils as those for
facial oils (see page 103) since the components are the same: a
high-quality carrier oil and essential oils. It is very easy to make a
body oil: fill an amber-colored bottle with 4 ounces of carrier oil,
and add 40 drops essential oils. Use the all-purpose oil recipe given
under "facial oils," or mix one of the following recipes. The
amount is always based on 4 ounces of carrier oil (3⅔ ounces of
almond oil or jojoba oil and ⅓ ounces of wheat germ oil).

For Normal Skin

> 10 rose
> 20 lavender
> 10 bergamot

For Irritated Skin

> jojoba oil
> 15 Roman chamomile
> 10 rose
> 15 geranium

For Mature Skin

> 15 frankincense
> 15 lavender
> 15 patchouli

For Oily Skin or Oily Seborrhea

> 15 cypress
> 15 cedarwood
> 15 frankincense

For Dry Skin

> 15 geranium
> 15 lavender
> 15 rosewood

Jojoba Body Lotion

The following recipe creates a body lotion that is very beneficial to the skin, providing it with moisture, smoothness, and a silky glow. A thin film of body lotion should always be applied after showering with hard tap water or swimming in chlorinated water in order to restore oil and moisture to the skin. (Hard tap water in combination with a strongly alkaline or synthetic soap will give rise to itching and a feeling of tension.)

Ingredients:

> 25 g anhydrous lanolin
> 25 g cocoa butter
> 125 g jojoba oil
> 50 g almond oil
> 25 g wheat germ oil
> 1 tbsp. vitamin E oil
> 50 drops essential oils
> Yield: about 10 oz.

Procedure:

Melt all ingredients except the essential oils in a double boiler until a clear liquid is obtained. Stir well. Pour the mixture into a bowl and stir slowly until it has cooled. Then add the essential oils, stir again, and pour into a container. This body oil rarely becomes rancid because of its high jojoba oil and wheat germ oil content. Use sparingly. It is suitable for all skin types.

Body Toner

Much like facial toner, body toner should refresh and stimulate the skin. It is best to make a large amount, fill a bottle with a spray top for immediate use, and store the rest in the refrigerator. Body toner has a very refreshing effect rubbed into the skin after a morning shower or an evening bath. Here are some suggestions:

Rosemary Toner

> 1 pint boiled water
> 2 oz. apple cider vinegar

20 rosemary
(cleansing and refreshing)

Flower Water Toner

1 pint rose water
a dash of apple cider vinegar
10 rosewood
10 bergamot
(astringent, cooling, calming)

Toner for Blemished, Oily Skin

½ pint pure (distilled) water
⅓ oz. pure grain alcohol
2–3 g borax or alum
20 geranium
10 lemon
(cleansing, disinfectant, astringent)

Sun Protection and Tanning Products

Sun Protection Cream

Ingredients:

40 g orange blossom water or aloe vera
40 g sesame oil or avocado oil
15 g anhydrous lanolin
5 g beeswax
20 lavender
Yield: about 4 oz.

Procedure:

Melt the beeswax and lanolin in a double boiler. Add vegetable oil and heat to 140°F. At the same time, warm flower water and aloe vera to the same temperature. Take both mixtures from the stove and gradually add the flower water or aloe vera to the oil while stirring slowly and constantly, until the mass is almost cold.

Then add the essential oil, stir again, fill into a container, and store in the refrigerator. Sesame oil has a medium sun-protection filter; aloe vera rejuvenates and heals (in the case of light burns). Lavender also heals and is an ideal oil to use for sunburn prevention.

Sun Protection Oil

This oil protects with lavender, sesame oil or avocado oil, and tans with carrot seed. It keeps the skin from drying out and doesn't have to be reapplied every time you go in the water.

Ingredients:

3⅔ oz. sesame oil or avocado oil
⅓ oz. wheat germ oil
1 tbsp. vitamin E oil
30 lavender
10 carrot seed
Yield: about 4 oz.

Procedure:

Fill all of the ingredients into an amber-colored bottle, shake well. Don't leave the oil out in the sun, as otherwise the essential oils become ineffectual.

Tanning Oil

This oil is to be used only for light to medium intensities of sunshine. Don't use it at a tanning studio or for strong natural sunshine. It keeps the skin from drying out.

Ingredients:

3⅔ oz. hazelnut oil
⅓ oz. wheat germ oil
30 bergamot
10 lemon
Yield: about 4 oz.

Procedure:

Pour ingredients into a dark bottle and shake well. Do not leave the bottle in the sun.

Tanning Lotion

This tanning lotion is a combination of substances that allow for a light tan and at the same time protect the skin from inflammation and sunburn.

Ingredients:

> 2 oz. distilled water
> 2 oz. witch hazel solution
> 20 bergamot
> 20 lavender
> Yield: about 4 oz.

Procedure:

Pour ingredients into an amber-colored bottle and shake well. Do not leave the bottle in the sun; store it in the refrigerator.

After-Sun Lotion

Use the all-purpose oil described under facial oils (see page 103) and add 40 drops lavender and 10 rose to 4 oz. oil.

After-Sun Bath

Add the following mixture to the bath water: 6 drops lavender, 4 drops carrot seed, 2 tablespoons jojoba oil, and 1 tablespoon honey.

In conclusion, here are a few recipes for hand, nail, foot, and mouth care:

Hand Care

Glycerine Gel for Dry, Chapped Hands

Ingredients:

> 3 tbsp. pectin or agar-agar
> 2 ½ oz. glycerine
> 2 ½ oz. witch hazel solution or aloe vera

6 tbsp. honey
15 Roman chamomile
10 lavender
Yield: about 6 oz.

Procedure:

Heat witch hazel solution or aloe vera in a doubler boiler. Dissolve the agar-agar or pectin in it and stir to make a homogeneous mixture. Remove from the heat, stir in glycerine, and let the mixture cool to 70°F. Finally, stir in the honey and essential oils. Let the mixture cool further without covering until the mass has jelled.

The gel can be thinned at any time by adding more liquid. To dissolve agar-agar, allow it to soften in a small amount for at least one hour and then heat and stir.

Hand-Washing Gel

This hand-washing gel is disinfectant, cleansing, and beneficial to the skin.

Ingredients:

10 oz. boiled water
4 oz. witch hazel solution
4 oz. glycerine soap or vegetable soap
2–3 tbsp. pectin
2 tbsp. honey
2 g borax (optional)
10 lavender
10 Roman chamomile
Yield: about 15 oz.

Procedure:

Heat water and witch hazel, sprinkle in the borax and stir, then add the soap and allow to melt. Heat about 2–3 cups of water separately beforehand, sprinkle pectin slowly into it, and stir until it has completely dissolved. Now add the pectin to the soap solution, stir, and let cool. When the mixture has reached skin temperature, add the honey and essential oils and stir again. For convenience, fill it into a bottle with a pump top.

After a few hours, the mixture will have jelled and is ready for use. If the gel has become too thick, it can be diluted with water. If it has become too thin, dissolve a little more pectin in warm water and add it, using as much pectin as is necessary to make the gel thicker. For particularly brittle, chapped hands and injured skin, use myrrh instead of lavender.

Hand-Care Oil

This very high-yielding, thick oil is recommended for dry, sore hands and after contact with aggressive substances.

Ingredients:

> 4 tbsp. lanolin
> 6 tbsp. olive oil or jojoba oil
> 10 Roman chamomile
> Yield: about 1½ oz.

Procedure:

Melt lanolin in double boiler until it is liquid; remove from heat, add olive oil, stir, and let cool. When the mixture is almost cool, add essential oil, stir again briefly, and fill into container.

Nail Care

Nail Care Oil

Ingredients:

> 1 oz. almond oil
> 2 lavender
> 2 sandalwood
> 2 cypress

Procedure:

Warm almond oil in a small bowl. Add oils and submerge the fingertips in the mixture for 10 minutes. The warm solution can then be applied to the toenails.

Nail Care Oil for Brittle Fingernails

Ingredients:

> 1 oz. vegetable oil
> 20 lemon

Procedure:

Pour the oils into a small amber-colored bottle, shake well, and apply to the nails on a regular basis.

Foot Treatments

Footbaths are good for the feet and promote general well-being. Even headaches can be treated with a refreshing peppermint bath. Heat about 2½ pints of water, pour into a bowl, and add one of the following mixtures:

For Sweaty Feet

> 3 lavender
> 3 sage
> *or*
> 3 clary sage
> 3 juniper
> 3 cypress
> *or*
> 6 pine

For Tired, Aching Feet

> 5 juniper
> 3 rosemary
> 2 lavender

For Headache

> 5 peppermint

Mouth Care

Mouthwash for Bad Breath

> 1 peppermint
> 1 thyme or bergamot
> 1 large glass (8 oz.) water
> (gargle, do not drink!)

Antiseptic Mouthwash

> 3 bergamot
> 2 lavender
> 1 large glass (8 oz.) water
> (gargle, do not drink!)

Mouthwash for Gum Care

> 1 pint pure water
> 3 tbsp. brandy
> 3 peppermint
> 3 thyme
> 3 fennel
> (gargle, do not drink!)

Recipes for Aromatic Baths

One of the most pleasant and effective methods for treating the skin is an aromatic bath. The combination of water, warmth, and the pleasant fragrance of the essences has several beneficial effects. Your skin is cleansed, treated, or healed with the essential oils, and at the same time is nourished and lubricated by other components such as vegetable oils—an important effect for normal, dry, and mature skin. In addition, inhalation of the stimulating scents affects one's mood and general well-being. Thus an aromatic bath (perhaps supplemented by music or even candlelight) can treat the mind as well as the body.

If a few drops of essential oil are added to water, most of it will simply float on the surface. In fact, some essential oils are more water soluble than others. In order to dissolve them evenly, it is best first to mix the essential oils with a carrier oil (e.g., jojoba, almond, or olive oil) and add when the bathtub is full. (You can naturally also put drops of the essences in the water.)

If you want your bath oil to disperse completely, add 1 teaspoon of Tween for every 4 ounces of carrier oil. Since Tween is not a vegetable substance, I myself do not use it; I simply accept the fact that oils will not completely disperse in water.

The vegetable oil will help to counter any drying effect of the harsh minerals in hot tap water; to soften the water, add 1 or 2 tablespoons of apple cider vinegar under the open faucet as the bath is filling. Other possible additives are whole milk, cream, and honey.

After an oil bath, the skin is soft and supple and has a moisture-protective cover. The result of bathing in hard water and with chemical bath additives is often tense, rough, itchy skin: if you suffer from one of these syndromes, pre-mix the essential oils with other natural additives in a cup, stir the mixture until smooth, and slowly pour into the bath water.

Occasional baths with nonirritating soap and apple cider vinegar are good for very oily skin. Please note that the presence of soap diminishes the effect of essential oils, preventing them from thoroughly penetrating and stimulating the skin. Cleansing baths with soap should therefore be taken without essential oils.

To prepare the skin for a treatment bath, start with a cleansing shower; the skin will then be better able to absorb the essences. Drape yourself in a towel and mix the bath oil while the tub is filling. (This might also be the ideal time to prepare a facial mask or pack.) Now get into the tub, relax, and breathe in the fragrance. From time to time, move the water around gently in order to spread the essential oils over your entire body. The skin will have absorbed the essential oils in about 15 to 20 minutes. If vegetable oil is added, a fine oil film will remain on the skin after the bath; this film should not be rubbed or showered off. Now apply a stimulating body toner or skin care oil. Wash off the facial mask, slip into a bathrobe, and let the oils continue to work. Your home will have the fragrance of essential oils and a pleasant atmosphere after the bath.

Any bath oil recipe can be increased by mixing about 4 ounces of carrier oil (jojoba, almond, or olive oil) with about 60 drops of essential oil. Keep the mixture in a dark bottle. This makes about 10 tablespoons of bath oil. Each bath calls for one tablespoon, or 1/3 ounce vegetable oil and 6 drops essential oils. Using these proportions, you can naturally prepare a mixture individually for each bath.

Consult the table on pages 44–46 for guidelines on mixing bath oils according to mood, physical state, or skin condition.

To prepare a child's skin care bath, take a small amount of a mild oil such as Roman chamomile, neroli, tangerine, orange, rose, or honey oil. These "children's oils" not only make the skin soft and heal little wounds, but also have very pleasant scents.

Please consult page 18 regarding possible irritation of sensitive skin and other restrictions in the use of certain oils.

Cleansing Baths
For All Skin Types

> 3 basil
> 3 rosemary
> 3 lemon
> (activates circulation, cleanses pores)

For Blemished and Tired Skin

> 6 sage
> 2 lemon
> 2 cups apple cider vinegar

Skin Care Baths
For Mature Skin

> 4 neroli
> 4 lavender
> 2 tbsp. honey
> 2 tbsp. avocado oil

For Oily Skin

6 basil
2 lemon
2 cups apple cider vinegar

For Dry Skin

6 carrot seed
6 bergamot
2 tbsp. vegetable oil
1 tbsp. honey

For Normal Skin

5 lavender
5 bergamot
2 tbsp. vegetable oil
1 tbsp. honey
  or
4 neroli
2 rose
1 cup whole milk
1 tbsp. honey
  or
3 ⅔ oz. almond oil
⅓ oz. wheat germ oil
¼ oz. vitamin E oil
20 Roman chamomile
20 lavender
(Makes enough to store a bottle in reserve)

Other Special Baths

Detoxification Bath

2 geranium
2 rosemary
2 juniper
2 lavender

Healing Bath for Blemished Skin

    6 tea tree
    6 lavender

Summer Bath Oil

    3 ⅔ oz. avocado oil or jojoba oil
    ⅓ oz. wheat germ oil
    40 lavender
    20 lemon
    (Makes enough to store a bottle in reserve)

After-Sun Bath

    6 lavender
    4 carrot seed
    2 tbsp. almond oil or jojoba oil

Sunburn Bath

    4 peppermint
    6 lavender
    2 tbsp. jojoba oil
    1 tbsp. honey

As a refreshing lotion after the bath, I recommend a mixture of 9 ounces of apple cider vinegar, 9 ounces of pure water, 10 drops of lavender, and 10 drops of rose. Place all ingredients in a bottle and shake well. To use, sprinkle on a washcloth and rub down the body. This lotion refreshes, cleanses, stimulates circulation, and is beneficial to the skin; it is very suitable for oily and blemished skin. Use less apple cider vinegar if its smell seems too strong.

Special Healing Recipes

The following healing recipes for illness, irritations, functional disturbances, and injuries of skin and tissue can be readily used without medical supervision. However, if improvement is not observed or if there is any doubt about the condition or treatment, please consult a doctor; even essential oils cannot perform miracles if medical guidance is needed.

In a *healing ointment*, the essential oils are particularly concentrated; this is what differentiates it from a skin care cream. The ointment is not absorbed quickly, but rather spreads a fine protective film on the surface of the skin. There the sebaceous film of the skin dissolves the essential oils so that they can penetrate deeply and develop their healing effects. A healing ointment should contain 2–3% essential oils. Use it only where necessary.

Mildly Inflamed Abscesses

Treat with hot compresses. Oils: bergamot, immortelle, lavender, Roman chamomile, garlic, or tea tree. Add about 15 drops to 2 pints of boiled hot water. The blend should always contain lavender. It calms swelling and inflammation and relieves pain. A mouth abscess can also be treated externally, but most effective is a mouth rinse with bergamot.

More Severely Inflamed, Reddish, Hot Abscesses

Treat with cold compresses. Oils: immortelle, onion. Add about 15 drops to 2 pints of cold water. This blend calms and heals inflammation.

Acne

Treat the spot with a special anti-inflammatory, antiseptic acne ointment. Add 90 drops of tea tree and 10 drops of lavender to jojoba healing ointment (see page 140). Apply the ointment mornings and evenings to clean skin. Be sure to use a skin care oil for acne (see recipe, page 106).

Athlete's Foot

Treat with lavender, myrrh, and/or tea tree. Mix 2 ounces of vegetable oil with 30 drops of lavender and 30 drops of myrrh, or with 40 drops of tea tree and 20 drops of lavender. This is a strong (3%) blend. Rub it into the afflicted areas mornings and evenings. (Put on socks at night.)

Blisters

Treat with undiluted lavender directly or applied to a sterile dressing or bandage. If the blister is wet or doesn't improve, use pure lavender and myrrh (1:1).

Bruises

Treat with ice-cold compresses (lavender, fennel, hyssop, or parsley). The blend should always contain lavender. Mix 2 pints of water with 15 drops essential oils. Use a skin oil or cream with rosemary afterward to stimulate circulation and dissolve the hematoma.

Calluses

Treat with garlic oil on a regular basis.

Cellulite

Treat cellulite with a skin oil and take a cellulite (hip) bath twice a week. The treatment should continue over a number of months and be supported by massage and exercise. Every activity promotes improvement.

Cellulite Massage Oil

> 2 oz. wheat germ oil
> 2 oz. jojoba oil
> *and*
> 10 geranium
> 20 orange
> 10 cypress
> *or*
> 10 geranium

10 orange
20 oregano

Cellulite Bath Mixture

5 juniper
3 orange
3 cypress
3 lemon
or
5 fennel
3 juniper
3 cypress
3 orange

Corns

Treat like warts (see page 139),with pure oils.

Eczema

Treat daily with a blend of 2 ounces of aloe vera, 20 drops of lavender, and 20 drops of immortelle or tea tree.

Healing of Scars

Mix a 2% healing oil from 4 ounces of jojoba oil or almond oil, 20 drops of neroli, 10 drops of lavender, 10 drops of bergamot, and 10 drops of frankincense. Or make an aloe vera healing ointment with the corresponding essential oils (see page 141). Apply daily, if possible before going to sleep.

Herpes

Dab lip blisters several times daily with pure melissa oils. Treat genital herpes with a base of jojoba healing ointment (see page 140) to which 20 drops of melissa and 5 drops of rose have been added. Take sitzbaths at regular intervals, using melissa and rose in a proportion of 6:4. Melissa is slightly irritating to the skin. This treatment also works well for shingles.

Inflammations of the Skin

Treat with healing oils or healing baths. Highly anti-inflammatory oils are benzoin, bergamot, eucalyptus, geranium, immortelle, blue chamomile, lavender, myrrh, peppermint, and tea tree. Mix 2 ounces of jojoba oil or aloe vera with 60 drops essential oils.

Pimples

Treat pimples locally with a base of jojoba healing ointment (see page 140) to which 30 drops of tea tree and 10 drops of lavender have been added. Apply the ointment to clean skin twice daily, mornings and evenings; or dab a few drops of undiluted tea tree, lavender, or lemon on the pimple.

Skin Fungus

Treat the affected skin areas daily with a blend of 2 ounces jojoba oil, 50 drops of tea tree *or* eucalyptus, and 20 drops of lavender (use smaller doses of essential oils for sensitive skin). If the skin fungus has spread to many areas of the body, aromatic baths with these oils are helpful.

Sunburn

See sunburn bath (page 134) and after-sun lotion (page 126).

Toenail Fungus

The probability of completely destroying this fungus is very limited since it is rooted deep in the nail bed. It can mainly just be prevented from spreading. Treat stubborn fungus with an alcohol–lavender–tea tree mixture or pure tea tree. (Note that alcohol dries out the skin.) Mix 2 ounces of pure grain alcohol with 20 drops of tea tree and 10 drops of lavender. Brush the mixture onto the nails, which have been cut as short as possible, mornings and evenings. After a week, continue to treat like athlete's foot, with an oil mixture.

Varicose Veins

Treat the legs daily with a blend of 4 ounces of almond oil, 40 drops of rosemary, 40 drops of cypress or juniper, and 20 drops of lemon. This is a strong (2%) mixture. Massage the legs with it, but never directly massage the varicose veins. Take a regular healing bath, covering only the legs with water and using a mixture of 6 drops of rosemary, 6 drops of cypress, and 4 drops of lemon. If lemon is not tolerated (in the case of sensitive skin), use juniper instead.

After the bath and massage, elevate the legs higher than the head and rest. As a supplement, take vitamins E and C, and eat generous amounts of garlic.

Warts

Apply 1 to 2 drops of undiluted lavender, garlic, clove, tea tree (eucalyptus as a substitute), thuja, or lemon oil daily. Cover the wart with a bandage afterward. Following successful treatment, healing can be promoted with wheat germ oil or vitamin E oil and lavender.

Weakness of the Connective Tissue

Treat the areas with a mixture of 2 ounces of jojoba oil, 2 ounces of wheat germ oil, 30 drops of rosewood, and 5 drops of rose. Massage the areas regularly with this skin oil.

Wounds, Sore Skin

Wounds and sore skin should be treated locally with a special healing oil, ointment, or lotion.

Wound Oil

Blend ½ ounce of jojoba oil and 5 drops of rose oil. This is an antiseptic oil with the healing and rejuvenating power of rose oil. Apply sparingly.

Wound Lotion

Mix 2 ounces of aloe vera with 15 drops of bergamot and 40 drops of lavender. A medium-strong mixture, it is disinfectant, anti-inflammatory, antiseptic, and promotes healing. Apply as a compress or bandage. In case of emergency, you can also use distilled water or boiled water blended with the essential oils.

Wound Cleanser

Wash wound with a mixture of distilled or boiled water (best with aloe vera added) and 2% tea tree. Use 15 drops of tea tree with ¾ ounce of water.

Wound Ointment

Here are three mixtures. The first is a light wound ointment that can be used in many situations and is simple to prepare. Warm 2 ounces of pretroleum jelly in a small glass container until it has become liquid. Then add 20 drops of bergamot or Roman chamomile, 20 drops of lavender, and 5 drops of tea (or eucalyptus). Stir well and store in a cool place. Since this ointment has a mineral oil base, it is not absorbed deeply by the skin.

For an ointment that is more readily absorbed, try a *jojoba healing ointment.* Here the healing power of jojoba oil and the essential oils complement each other.

Ingredients:

      2 oz. jojoba oil
      15 g beeswax
      40 drops essential oils
      Yield: about 2 ½ oz.

Procedure:

Heat the beeswax and jojoba oil in a double boiler until the mixture is clear. Then remove the mixture from the heat, stir well until it reaches skin temperature, and add 40 drops essential oils. Stir again and pour into a container. The consistency will thicken as it cools further.

This ointment is especially suitable for the treatment of scrapes, cuts, and burns; use 30 drops of lavender or Roman chamomile and 10 drops of bergamot for this purpose. Wounds that are not healing properly may be treated with jojoba healing ointment or with olive oil and lavender in a proportion of 10:1.

The following *aloe vera ointment* has even more healing power than the jojoba ointment, on which it is based.

Ingredients:

>   2 oz. jojoba oil
>   ½ oz. beeswax
>   .2 oz. cocoa butter
>   1½—2 oz. aloe vera
>   60 drops essential oils
>   Yield: about 4 ½ oz.

Procedure:

Melt the beeswax and cocoa butter in a double boiler. When the mixture becomes clear, add the jojoba oil and heat it to 140°F. The aloe vera should also be heated separately to 140°F. Take both mixtures from the heat and slowly add the aloe vera to the fat mixture while stirring constantly. Allow to cool until it reaches skin temperature, then add the essential oils and stir again. Place in a container and store in the refrigerator.

Note that the consistency of the ointment can be determined by the amount of aloe vera added. More than 1½ ounces of aloe vera will make the ointment thin and easy to spread. Finally, the same type of essential oils can be used here as are suggested for the jojoba healing ointment.

Recipes for Massage Oils

Along with proper skin care, regular massage of the body and face will effectively promote the skin functions and enhance skin beauty. The cornified upper layer of the skin is rubbed away in the process of massage, which in turn stimulates the breathing of the skin and cell rejuvenation. The skin thereby becomes more receptive to the effects of skin care cosmetics and healing substances. Another beneficial effect of massage is its stimulation of removal of waste products and detoxification of the body.

A body massage should use a nutritive and stimulating body oil, which can be prepared from a carrier oil (almond, jojoba, avocado, or wheat germ) blended with essential oils. (The fragrance table that begins on page 45 can provide many suggestions for possible scents.)

Essential oils can be chosen either by "following your nose"— that is, simply picking whatever smells good at the moment—or by aiming for a particular physical and/or emotional reaction by choosing oils according to their known effects. In most cases, the oil whose fragrance you prefer will also be the one that is right for your physical and emotional balance.

The spectrum of effects from a massage is very wide. It provides general physical and mental stimulation; the nerves are relaxed, the emotions balanced, the mood lightened, and fears, troubles, and worries are chased away. When used along with a massage, essential oils can also stimulate circulation, tone muscles and skin, and relieve muscle pain, rheumatism, tired legs, cellulite, and the like.

It is simple to make a massage oil. Blend about 40 drops essential oils with 4 ounces of vegetable oil, always adding about ⅓ ounce of wheat germ oil to prevent the oxidation of the blend as long as possible (a step that is unnecessary if jojoba oil is used). Pour the contents into an amber-colored bottle, shake well—and the massage oil is ready.

Don't be confused by the term "massage oil." In fact, any body oil or moisturizing lotion with an oil base can be used as a massage oil. Consult the section on essential oils (pages 23–44) and the corresponding table (page 44) to develop your own blends. To make a massage oil that also doubles as a skin care oil, use the essential oils which correspond to your skin type (see page 82). The following recipes are all based on 4 ounces of carrier oil:

Massage Oil for Psychological Well-being

Stimulating Oil

>   25 rosewood
>   10 geranium
>   10 geranium
>   5 orange

Relaxing Oil

>   20 lavender
>   15 clary sage
>   5 melissa

To Combat Stress, Depression

>   20 ylang-ylang
>   10 patchouli
>   10 jasmine

Body-Function Massage Oils

Weakness of the Connective Tissue

>   2 oz. wheat germ oil
>   40 lavender

Tired, Aching Legs

>   20 rosemary
>   15 lavender
>   5 peppermint

Cellulite

Jojoba or wheat germ oil
20 orange
20 cypress
10 sage

To Tauten the Skin

25 lavender
5 neroli
5 rose
5 frankincense

To Promote Weight Loss

20 juniper
15 cypress
5 rosemary
(apply only to fatty areas; a generally stimulating mixture)

To Increase Breast Size

15 ylang-ylang
15 geranium
(must be used daily for a number of months)

Skin Care Oil

3 oz. jojoba oil or almond oil
½ oz. arnica oil
⅓ oz. wheat germ oil
20 rosewood
10 geranium
10 orange
(promotes circulation, rejuvenates, activates, smooths and
   nourishes the skin)

The Natural Massage

To begin a massage properly, start with the feet, our point of contact with the earth. By massaging the reflex zones of the feet, it is possible to stimulate all the organs without touching them directly. For this reason, the feet should be massaged frequently—not only when they are tired or aching. Regular foot massage is especially recommended for those whose work forces them to be on their feet much of the time.

After a relaxing or refreshing foot bath with lavender or peppermint, give the feet a strong massage by rubbing, kneading, and tapping them, and running the knuckles of the hand from the toes to the balls of the feet. A reaction of pain here and there is a completely normal indication that a reflex zone is reacting or a muscle is cramped. Finally, using the pressure of both hands with slightly spread fingers, draw lines on the tops of the feet from the toes to the ankles.

Now go to the *ankles* and *calves* and massage them from bottom to top. If you have varicose veins, never massage the veins directly. You can knead the thighs, if they are not sensitive to pain, more intensely, and slap them with the palms of the hands.

Please treat the *belly* more gently. Below the navel is the *hara*, or life center. When this center is stimulated, we receive vital energy and simultaneously attain a state of great rest, which is reflected as outer beauty in the relaxed facial muscles. With both hands, stroke the area around the navel in a clockwise direction. Do this about sixty times. If you hear digestive noises, then you have stimulated your intestines, and good digestion is important for pure skin! We all gain weight most quickly in the belly. To distribute excess fat, vigorously knead any bulges and move them to all sides.

Next, a vigorous *breast* massage strengthens the connective tissue and stimulates the circulation. This prevents the breasts from becoming slack. Massage them vigorously with both hands in a clockwise direction. If you think your breasts are too small, a special massage oil can be applied (see page 144). Be sure to lightly pull and knead the nipples (particularly inverted nipples).

It is best to massage the *neck* with dry, spread fingers by drawing lines from the collar bone to the chin and up to the ears.

The *facial massage* is most beneficial after a steam bath. Use a special facial oil or facial cream. With clean fingertips, rhythmically tap the entire face as if it were a drum. This stimulates the meridians in your face. To avoid getting a double chin, press the bent thumb deeply under the jaw bone a number of times. (Shiatsu therapists say that a reaction of pain here is a sign that a person eats too much.) Now put both hands on the cheeks and evenly push the muscles and tissue back and forth in a clockwise direction and then counterclockwise.

Next vigorously massage the side of the nose back and forth with the index and middle fingers. This stimulates not only the skin but also the digestion, since the stomach meridian runs through this area. In addition, you can also draw lines with the fingertips, as shown in figure 3. Do all of these massages very gently on mature skin.

A gentle *eye* massage will leave the eyes relaxed and clear. Massage this area carefully so that no oil gets in the eyes. Put the index and middle fingers on the eyes so that the fingertips touch the forehead bone and move around the eyeball with gentle circular motions. Afterward, let the fingers rest lightly on the closed eyes.

The concluding massage of the *head* can be done with a refreshing hair lotion (peppermint or rosemary). Massage the scalp in strong circular motions: this will increase blood circulation in the head and is very invigorating. A head massage is particularly recommended for mature skin.

For a final revitalizing exercise, lie down at an angle with the feet elevated higher than the head. This increases the blood circulation in the head and face and accelerates the metabolism, and the nutrients reach the scalp more quickly. Twenty minutes of rest in this position will be more refreshing than an hour of lying flat.

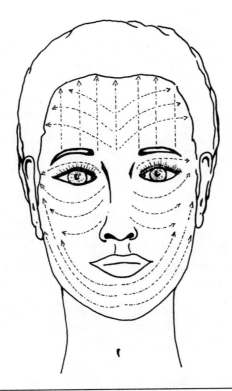

Figure 3: Schematic for rejuvenating facial massage

Shiatsu Massage for Beauty

Some cosmetic schools now offer Shiatsu massage in addition to cosmetic treatment. (Acupuncturists also draw on the methods of Shiatsu to treat skin diseases and blemished skin.) The word *Shiatsu* comes from Japanese (*shi* = finger; *atsu* = pressure). This centuries-old oriental method of massage is a preferred form of therapy in Japan, where there are thousands of practicing Shiatsu therapists.

Shiatsu is based upon the stimulation of acupressure or acupuncture points (*tsubos*) that lie on the so-called meridian lines, the fourteen channels through which our energy flows. The meridians or energy channels are named after the organs or body systems, such as the stomach, large intestine, small intestine, gall bladder, cardiovascular system, kidneys, liver, bladder, and so forth. The Shiatsu therapist can influence various symptoms by applying pressure to any of 361 *tsubos*. (Neither the *tsubos* nor the meridian lines are visible.)

To understand how Shiatsu works, we must be aware that the body is a closed system in which every function is dependent upon another function. For example, if we do not properly digest our food—a process for which the intact functioning of spleen and stomach is necessary—then our skin does not receive sufficient nourishment. By the same token, when waste products remain too long in the large intestines, the body (and thus the skin) will gradually be affected by the toxins thus retained. The same applies in the case of limited functioning of the kidneys, small intestines, liver, and gall bladder, the other important organs involved in detoxification. The lungs are detoxification organs as well, and provide our blood with the oxygen necessary for proper skin functioning. All of these organs can be influenced through acupressure and acupuncture points, and their improved functioning eventually also benefits the skin.

Since many meridians run through the face and are easily located, I have chosen some "beauty points" related to the condition of the skin and the facial muscles that can be stimulated in home treatment. With regular Shiatsu treatment, you are certain to notice improvement or harmonization of your body functions and your skin. All points are to be stimulated with an extended index finger, middle finger, or thumb, or with a smooth, dull object, three times for 5–7 seconds each through pressure in an inward direction. The pressure should not create pain, but should be noticeable.

Point 1 lies at about the middle of a line extending between the eyebrows along the middle of the head. It is stimulated to promote hair growth and to soothe headaches and nervous tension.

Point 2, known as "the sun," lies on the temples at the hair line. It is stimulated to soothe headaches and red, swollen eyes.

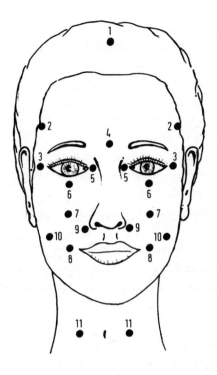

Figure 4: Acupuncture points for facial massage

Point 3 is located about one third of an inch from the outer end of the corner of the eye, in a recess on the gallbladder meridian. It is stimulated for headaches and eye problems.

Point 4 lies between the eyebrows. It is stimulated for headaches, stuffy nose, and facial tension in this area.

Point 5 lies deep in the corner of the eye (push up into the recess with the finger). It is located on the bladder meridian and called "Bright Light." It is pressed to help swollen, tired eyes and for concentration and inner collection.

Point 6 lies directly under the pupil, in the recess on the cheek-bone (on the stomach meridian), and is stimulated for facial pain and tension, stuffy nose, and digestive disturbances.

Point 7 is about the width of two fingers below point 6 in a small recess at the end of the cheekbone (on the stomach meridian). Stimulate it for about 15 seconds to relieve facial pain or tensions and frontal sinusitus.

Point 8 lies some distance from the outer end of the corner of the mouth, below point 7 on the stomach meridian. It is pressed when the facial muscles are tense and there is stomach pain.

Point 9 is located next to the nostrils in a small recess on the meridian of the large intestine. It is stimulated for facial muscle tension, stuffy nose, and colds.

Point 10 lies in a little hollow on the jaw joint when the jaw is tensed. It is located on the stomach meridian and should be pressed for pain in the teeth.

Point 11 is located next to the larynx on a major artery (on the stomach meridian) and stimulates the thyroid gland and the production of hormones that promote beauty. In addition, the blood pressure is lowered when you gently press this point for 10 to 15 seconds.

Note that most of these points are found on both sides of the face, the right side as well as the left. Press both points at the same time. On the forehead, just behind the hairline, are further beauty points. Take these points into consideration when you are massaging the head.

5 🌿 Hair Care

Structure and Functions of the Hair

Many thousands of years ago, the bodies of our ancestors were entirely covered with thick hair which protected them against the elements and dirt. Once clothing was adopted, this protective hair gradually disappeared, leaving the scalp the only area to be still extensively covered.

Healthy hair is slightly oily, light, strong, constantly self-renewing, and easy to comb. It reacts to the foods you eat, and these in turn should provide the hair with the minerals and vitamins it needs in order to grow properly. These essential substances should not just be taken as pills. Hormonal changes, hereditary factors, and psychological burdens also play an important role in the health of our hair. Overexposure to ultraviolet rays, pollutants in the air, or other toxic substances; ingestion of alcohol, nicotine, and chlorinated water; illness anywhere in the body and the side effects of medication; lack of scalp massage and the use of nylon brushes—all change and impair the condition of the hair. You do not have to accept such changes as an inevitable fact of life, however.

151

Our hair is just as sensitive as our skin. The structure and fullness of the hair are dependent upon its coloring. Blond hair is fine; dark hair and red hair are more coarse. Blonds have the most hair (about 140,000 hairs), redheads the least (about 90,000). One square inch of scalp contains approximately 720 hairs, each of which grows .01 inches in a month's time and can live two to three years. Then a new hair or a new root is formed in the same spot. We lose about eighty hairs a day. To remove old, dead hair and stimulate the natural growth, you must brush your hair regularly and intensively. But please, to avoid static electricty, not with a nylon brush! In the old days, one hundred strokes with a brush was recommended to remove the old hair, massage the scalp, and stimulate the circulation. But even without counting strokes, a thorough brushing twice a day can save you from spending excessive time at the hairdresser's and wasting money on expensive hair-care products.

The hair grows out of the scalp, while the skin contains the hair root, the erector pili muscle, the sebaceous gland, the blood vessel, and the hair shaft (see figure 2, page 72). The erector pili muscle determines the direction in which the hair lies. The sebaceous gland provides the oily substance sebum, which coats the hair, giving it suppleness and strength and protecting it from ultraviolet radiation, dirt, and unfavorable atmospheric conditions. Every time hair moves (for example, when it is brushed or combed), sebum from the sebaceous glands is brought to the surface and the blood vessels brings it the substances vital for life. Since the hair is made of keratin cells, which consist almost exclusively of protein, it is particularly important to supply it with protein in the form of milk products, fish, soy products, nuts, seeds, and the essential fatty acids contained in cold-pressed vegetable oils.

Care of the Hair

Hair is an important element in appearance. Yet we wash, cut, blow-dry, dye, curl, tone, spray, and style it, to the point that we really should feel sorry for it. The market is flooded with products for washing, toning, and conditioning the hair, all containing a vast assortment of substances to guarantee healthy, strong, shiny, elastic, easy-to-style hair with natural hold, as well as preparations which supposedly fight dandruff, split ends, and hair loss. Are all these products really needed?

What is needed, first of all, is periodic shampooing. This washing process should remove dirt, hair scales, and extra fat from the hair. The active substances in most shampoos accomplish that much. But all active substances, even good old soap, attack the acid mantle of the scalp and wash away the hair's oil film. In addition, the aggressive synthetic substances in cheap shampoos damage the upper layer of the skin and the hair follicles. The scalp dries out, the hair becomes like straw and falls out. Once the hair has lost its natural protection, it becomes dirty more quickly, the sebaceous glands are stimulated to increase production of sebum, and finally the hair becomes oily, so that it must be treated with still another product—a vicious circle, but one that is highly profitable for the cosmetic industry!

The spectrum of active substances in shampoos allows for all sorts of possibilities: one washes away all the oil, the other more dirt and less oil, and so on. Hence the need to label shampoos specifically "for oily hair" or "for dry hair." The effect of chemical and mineral substances in all synthetic hair shampoos is altogether too strong. Their alkaline substances do make the hair fluffier, but only for a short time before it collapses again. You probably have observed how after washing your hair in the morning, you have a light and attractive hairstyle. After several hours, the hair has flattened unbecomingly against the head. In order to reduce their negative effects on the scalp, shampoos that are mildly alkaline or pH neutral are now tempered by the addition of citric acid, for example.

After each washing, hair should be rinsed with an acidic substance, no matter what kind of shampoo is used. Lemon juice, natural apple cider vinegar, milk, and beer are all suited for this purpose—to remove the detergent and calcium residue and restore the acid equilibrium of the scalp. A few drops of essential oil can be added to give the hair a pleasant scent. Their effect on the scalp continues even after the rinse. Fine and soft hair should only be given a quick rinse.

A hair lotion, highly recommended for all types of hair—particularly when functional disturbances of the scalp and hair roots are present—should be massaged into the slightly damp hair. It has a good effect on the scalp and hair roots, as well as a pleasant fragrance.

Functional Disturbances of the Hair and Scalp

When we consider the effects caused by the aggressive chemical agents used in permanents, dyeing, toning, and styling, it is a wonder that some people still have hair on their heads. For example, the hair's natural seal is dissolved with sulfur compounds so that the hair can be shaped as desired, or chemical dyes are poured over the scalp and absorbed by the hair shaft. Naturally the result is hair that is dry, brittle, dull, slack, and greatly in need of additional care—and the ultimate cost may be loss of hair at a later date.

The functional disturbances ssuch as dandruff, itching, or rashes on the scalp that plague us occasionally can be the result of aggressive hair-washing. It is best to first try changing shampoos. Itching and rashes can be treated with hair lotion to which essential oils have been added. The hair lotion is then actually a scalp-massage lotion.

Dandruff itself—the flaking of dead cells from the scalp—is normal; the problem is one of degree. You can counteract the increased discharge of flakes by regulating skin functions. Massage and stimulating essential oils will activate the metabolism, but as far as increased washing is concerned, the opinions of the experts vary greatly. Some recommend a daily shampoo for dandruff, others limit it to no more than twice a week. My own experience has shown that frequent washing with much soap stimulates the production of sebum, which makes the hair oily that much more quickly and causes the protective film of the skin to lose its equilibrium. Still, it's important to find out what works best for you.

Treatment of Hair Types and Hair Problems with Essential Oils

Normal Hair

Normal hair can be cared for with Roman chamomile, carrot seed, lavender, clary sage, rosewood, sage, thyme, rosemary, cedarwood, lemon, or cypress. Roman chamomile and lemon can be used to color light hair, and rosemary and rosewood to color dark hair. Try an occasional hair treatment with one or more of these essential oils in a base of almond oil or jojoba oil.

Oily Hair

Use clary sage, juniper, cedarwood, or cypress to care for oily hair. An occasional jojoba treatment will be useful as well.

Dry Hair

Use geranium, lavender, or juniper to care for dry hair, since these stimulate the sebaceous glands to restore the hair to its natural oiled condition. A periodic hair treatment with these oils is particularly beneficial for dry hair; you can also use the oils listed above under "Normal Hair" for the treatment.

Dandruff

For dandruff, eucalyptus, lavender, clary sage, patchouli, peppermint, rosemary, sage, tea tree, juniper, cypress, or cedarwood can be used in shampoos, rinses, and hair oils. Treat the hair with olive oil or jojoba oil on a regular basis. Rinses, hair lotions, and scalp massages with apple cider vinegar and peppermint or one of the other oils listed above can be very helpful.

Hair Loss

For hair loss, the hair should be washed and cared for with products containing cajeput, clary sage, peppermint, rosemary, sage, thyme, or cedarwood. After rinsing, a hair lotion containing the same oil should be massaged well into the scalp. Avocado oil and aloe vera will stimulate hair growth and should be used as a treatment on a regular basis.

Split, Brittle Hair

Damaged hair and split ends should be given regular treatments. Use packs and oil treatments with warm jojoba oil, lanolin, or burdock root oil.

See the following table for an overview of oils used in hair-care preparations.

Recipes for Hair Care

Washing the Hair

Hair care starts with washing the hair. Use a natural shampoo with a pH value of 4–6 for this purpose. Aromatic shampoos are best created by blending essential oils in a shampoo without synthetic agents. Simply add 1–2% of any essential oils corresponding to your hair type to the shampoo and shake well.

You can also make your own shampoo from scratch. Essential oils, water, and soft soap can be combined to create a hair-care product that provides your hair with shine, stimulates the scalp, and

Essential Oils for Hair Care	brittle hair	dandruff	dark hair	dry hair	hair loss	light hair	normal hair	oily hair	split ends
Bergamot								•	
Birch				•					
Burdock Root	•								•
Cajeput				•					
Carrot seed				•			•		
Cedarwood		•		•			•	•	
Chamomile, Roman						•	•		
Clary Sage		•					•	•	
Cypress							•	•	
Eucalyptus		•							
Frankincense				•					
Geranium				•					
Jojoba oil	•								
Juniper								•	
Lavender oil				•			•	•	
Lemon						•	•		
Patchouli		•							
Rosemary		•	•		•		•		
Rosewood			•				•		
Sage					•		•		
Sandalwood			•						
Tea Tree		•							
Thyme					•		•		

regulates the production of sebum. People once shampooed with rainwater; today it is recommended that you use distilled water, boiled water, or bottled spring water.

When using synthetic shampoos, always rinse afterward in order to remove the residue of detergent from the base of the hair. Even when homemade soap shampoos—such as those described in these pages—are used, a rinse is advisable to wash out any residue of soap or calcium from the hair. At the same time, it stabilizes the acid equilibrium of hair and skin. The hair feels pleasantly soft after a rinse.

Basic Shampoo

Ingredients:

> 1 cup liquid soap
> ½ cup water
> ½ tbsp. vegetable oil (jojoba, olive, avocado)
> 10 drops essential oil

Procedure:

Pour all ingredients into a bottle with a spray top and shake lightly. (First put in the water, then the soap, since the mixture otherwise foams too much.) Choose from the essential oils recommended on page 157 for this mixture. To simultaneously treat the hair and stimulate the scalp, use 5 drops of lavender and 5 drops of peppermint. Apply only a little of this shampoo, since it has a high yield. The vegetable oil restores fat to the hair, which then feels soft and doesn't dry out. If your hair is often exposed to strong sun, the amount of vegetable oil can be increased. You don't need a conditioner after washing your hair with this shampoo. For seborrhea, hair loss, and/or dandruff, replace the water with aloe vera and be sure to use jojoba oil.

Hair-wash Gel with Aloe Vera

Ingredients:

> 25 oz. pure water or spring water
> 2 oz. liquid soap
> 2 oz. aloe vera
> 2 tbsp. pectin
> 20 drops of essential oil
> Yield: about 29 oz.

Procedure:

Boil the water, then add the soft soap, and let this mixture simmer for about thirty minutes. Dissolve the pectin in 2–3 cups of this mixture and stir thoroughly, making sure that no lumps form. Now add the pectin solution, the aloe vera, and the essential oils to the original soap solution and pour it all into a bottle with a spray top. Or divide the gel between two bottles and keep the reserve bottle in the refrigerator.

After several hours, the hair-wash gel will have thickened and be ready for use. If it isn't thick enough, add a bit more dissolved pectin to it and shake the bottle well. If it has become too thick, add some water. Instead of aloe vera, lavender water can be used: aloe vera stimulates hair growth, while lavender reduces the production of sebum, making it particularly suitable for oily hair. Look under "Hair Types and Problems" (page 155) to find the appropriate essential oils for your homemade shampoo.

Rinses

After washing the hair, rinse it thoroughly with an aromatic water and dry it with a towel. The hair will then have a pleasant scent. Rosewood or rosemary used over a longer period of time will impart a silky, dark shimmer to the hair. A somewhat lighter color results from applications of lemon oil, lemon juice, or chamomile. To make the rinse, use about 10–15 drops essential oils corresponding to hair type in 2 pints of boiled water or spring water. Here are two special recipes:

Basic Rinse

Ingredients:

> 5 oz. boiled water or spring water
> 2 oz. apple cider vinegar
> 10–15 drops essential oils
> Yield: 7 oz.

Shine Rinse
Ingredients:

> 1 pint apple cider vinegar or lemon juice
> 1 pint boiled water or spring water
> 25 drops rosemary/rosewood (for dark hair) or
> Roman chamomile (for light hair)
> Yield: about 2 pints

Procedure:

Mix ingredients well in a spray-top bottle. The recipe features a strong concentration of apple cider vinegar, whose scent you will have to like (or at least not mind). But since the rinse is washed out of the hair and the scent of the vinegar quickly vanishes, you don't have to worry about smelling like a pickle. The amount is enough to rinse short hair many times. Massage well into the hair and wash it out quickly. The rinse removes calcium and soap residue, activates and stimulates the scalp, and is suitable for oily hair, dandruff, and itching of the scalp. If the itching is very intense, use peppermint.

Hair Tonic

To balance any hair care program, a hair tonic can be massaged in and left on the hair. It imparts a pleasant fragrance and continues to affect the scalp for many hours. Hair tonic should particularly be used for dandruff, oily hair, and itching of the scalp. It is made like the rinse. To 1 pint of water, add 20–25 drops essential oils. Use peppermint for scalp itching; rosemary for dandruff; and lavender, clary sage, juniper, cedarwood, or cypress for oily hair. Add ½ pint aloe vera to combat hair loss and seborrhea of the scalp. Apple cider vinegar (in a proportion of about 10% of the hair tonic) may be added for oily hair and dandruff.

Hair Tonic for Dandruff and Oily Hair
Ingredients:

> 15 oz. boiled water or spring water

2 oz. apple cider vinegar
10 lavender
10 clary sage

Hair Tonic for Seborrhea, Hair Loss, Insufficient Growth

Ingredients:

½ pint boiled water or spring water
½ pint aloe vera
15 clary sage
10 rosemary

Activating Hair Tonic

Ingredients:

1 pint boiled water or spring water
10 peppermint
10 rosemary (dark hair) or
10 Roman chamomile (light hair)
(refreshing, stimulating, deodorizing)

Setting Lotion

Honey added to the hair tonic sculpts the hair. Generally, 2–3 tablespoons of honey to a pint of water are sufficient. The water must be warm in order to dissolve the honey, but do not use boiling water, since the active ingredients of the honey will then be destroyed.

With the help of the summary of essential oils for hair care along with the summary of fragrances you can choose "your own scent." Instead of rosemary, for example, you might use the wood scents, which men generally prefer (e.g., sandalwood and cedarwood). Or for dandruff a woman might also use patchouli, which would be harmonized with the scent of her facial cosmetics or perfume. Creating hair care products with essential oils affords many possibilities to play with the fragrances.

Hair Treatments

An occasional hair treatment both nourishes and grooms the hair, particularly if the hair is washed frequently and has been exposed to sun, wind and salt water or chlorinated water. If you have the feeling that your hair has become dry, thin, straw-like, brittle, dandruffy, and split, an oil treatment will work wonders for it. Even oily hair needs nutrients and should be treated with oil. This makes for a more balanced sebum production, better circulation, and deep cleansing of the base of the hair.

Jojoba oil is particularly suited for this purpose, since it is effective against dandruff and split ends. Olive oil also works well by stimulating hair growth and providing the scalp with proteins and vitamins.

The following recipes are based on 2 oz. of vegetable oil. This amount is sufficient to treat short hair a number of times and very long hair once. The oil, which should be warmed in advance, is mixed with 20–25 drops essential oil and thoroughly massaged into the freshly washed, slightly damp hair. While the treatment is working, cover the hair with a plastic shower cap and a large towel. This keeps the head and oil warm, preventing the active ingredients from evaporating. If you have the opportunity and the weather is good, sit in the sun. Leave the oil treatment on normal hair for up to an hour, up to 2 hours in cases of inadequate growth or other functional disturbances. Then wash the hair first with only warm water, followed by a shampoo. Here are several mixtures:

For Normal Dark Hair

> 10 lavender
> 10 rosewood or cedarwood

For Normal Light Hair

> 15 Roman chamomile
> 5 lemon

For Oily Hair

> 8 bergamot

8 cypress
8 lavender

For Dandruff

Jojoba oil
10 eucalyptus or tea tree
15 rosemary

For Dry Hair

15 lavender
10 geranium

For Hair Loss

Avocado oil or olive oil
8 rosemary
8 sage
8 cedarwood or lavender
(optional: add 1 tbsp. burdock root oil)

For Brittle Hair and Split Ends

Jojoba oil or olive oil
1 tbsp. vitamin E oil
20 drops essential oils (according to hair color and
    condition)

Hair Packs

An alternative to an oil treatment is the hair pack: according to
how thick your hair is, mix jojoba oil or avocado oil with 2 to
4 egg yolks and 20 drops of essential oil, according to your hair
color, type, or problem. Massage the pack in well and cover the
hair so that it is airtight. After 30 minutes, wash it out first with
water alone, then shampoo well, followed by a rinse.

6 🌿 Natural Perfumes

Perfume and Its Effects

Let us now turn to the most stimulating facet of essential oils—their use as perfume. Why do we actually use perfumes? What is the effect of their exquisite fragrance? For thousands of years people have enveloped themselves in pleasant scents. They bathe in sweet-smelling essences, use perfumed soaps, and pamper the body with fragrant oils, creams, and ointments.

The use of a perfume is meant to stimulate our own sense of smell as well as that of other people. Like a flower that exudes its scent in order to attract insects, we perfume ourselves in order to attract someone else's attention. We all know what it means to feel drawn toward someone because of the scent that radiates from them. Perfume should therefore evoke the sense of freshness, sympathy, attraction, and pleasure in others. We then influence their feelings and decisions.

Body odor can be covered up or enhanced and made more pleasant with perfume. This is a matter of very specific, fine nuances of body scent. However, extremely strong and unpleasant perspiration tends to become intensified by the use of perfume. Most commercially available perfumes use aphrodisiac, or sexually-stimulating, fragrances to arouse the pleasure center so that others experience us as attractive and likeable. The aphrodisiac fragrances are mostly derived from blossoms (lilac, rose, ylang-ylang, neroli, jasmine, tuberose, violet, mimosa, narcissus, orchid, etc.) and other plant elements (patchouli, sandalwood, cardamon, pepper, and cinnamon), or are synthesized chemically. Clary sage also has a euphoric, stimulating effect and contributes to relaxation. Orange and tangerine could also be added to the list since they make us feel light, relaxed, and happy—an important prerequisite for erotic mood-setting.

The use of flower oils seems fairly obvious. Blossom fragrances are very intense; they attract insects that carry the pollen to other flowers and thus assure reproduction. The blossom scents are just as stimulating to our own pleasure centers.

The perfume industry also uses animal secretions and their synthetic imitations. Among these are civet (from cats caged on farms), musk (from the musk deer, which lives in Tibet, Nepal, and China), and ambergris (a rarely-found secretion of the whale, a by-product of whaling). Yet the fragrances that can be derived from plants are so diverse and abundant that we can do without imprisoning and killing animals.

Natural Body Odors and Their Function in Perfume

Individual body scent is created by approximately one million sweat glands in the hairy parts of the body (head, armpits, genital area) and is most intensely noticed in those parts. The perspiration of the remaining body parts has almost no scent of its own, but will take on the odor various of foods or drinks soon after they are ingested. The best known examples of this are garlic and alcohol.

The hairy areas of the body all contain many saturated fatty acids. In addition, the armpits and genital area have bacteria on the skin. These bacteria determine the individual scent of those areas. The intensity of scent ranges from mild in the head area to pungent in the armpits. Body scent generally is most intensive in the evening and at night, when the body temperature rises and there is an increase in perspiration. The fragrance of perfume is therefore also stronger in the evening and at night since the aroma evaporates more quickly and mixes with the more intense body scent.

Corresponding to hair coloring, three primary types of body odors can be distinguished based upon the respective skin constitution and metabolic characteristics. Blonds have a sour and cheesy scent, redheads have a sharp and acrid scent, while dark-haired people have a sweet-pungent scent reminiscent of perspiration. A mixture of all of these scents in their natural intensity can be very erotic.

The makers of perfume aim at creating a mixture similar to the body scent so that it can optimally develop its sexually-stimulating effect in harmony with the other scents contained in the perfume. The following essential oils have an erotic effect with scents similar to those of the body, and are suitable for use in an aphrodisiac perfume:

> *Indole*, which can be found in neroli, jasmine, tuberose, lilac, and other blossom scents, as well as their synthetic imitations, has an animalistic character that is subtly reminiscent of human secretions. In fact we find this scent in almost all classical perfumes (such as "Shalimar").
>
> *Frankincense*, the scent of which corresponds to the perspiration and body odor of dark-haired and red-haired people.
>
> *Myrrh*, the scent of which is similar to the perspiration and body odor of blond-haired people.
>
> *Carrot seed* and *geranium*, the scent of which corresponds to the slightly sour scent of blonds.
>
> *Musk* is derived from hibiscus plant *(H. abelmoschus)* seeds, also called ambretta. This is the plant counterpart to animal musk.

Its character is animalistic, corresponding to the general scent of the body and its excretions.

Amber or styrax of the amber tree *Liquidambar orientalis* is an oil with an aphrodisiac, sweet-flowery scent; this scent corresponds to that of the head and pubic hair of dark-haired people.

Cypress (when free of turpentine) corresponds to the scent of the pubic hair and body odor of blonds.

Be forewarned that pure musk and amber are very expensive. Amber or musk offered inexpensively in the form of oils or resins are mixtures made of different scents that combine into the same smell.

The oils that are absolutely *not* aphrodisiac are angelica root, lemon, eucalyptus, petitgrain, peppermint, spearmint, rosemary, spike lavender, verbena, basil, and juniper. These fresh scents primarily remind us of purity and cleanliness. Some perfumes similarly impart a bright, clear scent, giving the feeling of freshness which is considered important today. Perfumed laundry detergents, dishwashing liquids, bath salts, bubble bath, and soaps are all examples of products that mostly feature the scents of lemon, lime, or pine. They make us feel pure and fresh.

Unpleasant body odors should be remedied not with perfume but rather with a deodorant (deodorized soap, deodorant stick or lotion). Deodorizing scents either block the production of perspiration or neutralize unpleasant body odors. Women have more apocrine sweat glands than men do and are generally more attentive to this problem. Unfortunately, the products available are so strong that they often irritate the skin and even damage clothing—side effects that can be avoided by either simply accepting your body scent or mixing a deodorizing natural body oil. The typical scents of deodorants are very refreshing and quick to evaporate. These include bergamot, citronella, eucalyptus, lemongrass, petitgrain, peppermint, pine, rosemary, thyme, and cypress.

In my experience, our spirits are more gently and pleasantly stimulated by essential oils in unadulterated perfume than by synthetic perfumes. With time and experience in working with essential oils, you will develop a feeling for the difference between their natural scents and those of cheap synthetic perfumes. You will also be astonished at how your sense of smell refines so that you perceive many more fragrances than before.

Only the most adventurous readers will try to create a perfume sophisticated enough to meet all the requirements of a classical perfume. Yet for those who love to experiment, this little excursion into the world of perfumes may encourage you not only to create functional cosmetics, but also to allow them a definite scent—exotic, erotic, fresh, or flowery. As the person who wears the cosmetics, you are the one who will ultimately encounter it most—and you should enjoy it.

Commercially Manufactured Perfumes

Today's ready-made perfumes contain up to two hundred different and almost exclusively synthetic fragrances. Yet although many scents have already been synthetically imitated, an *absolute* imitation of flower oils has not been achieved. Commercial perfumes are also much too expensive, considering what the manufacturers pay for the raw materials. The fragrances are suspended in an alcohol or alcohol-water solution with fixatives. (A fixative is a substance with a heavy molecular weight and a high boiling point. In contrast to the essential or synthetic oils, it rarely evaporates and thereby also prevents their speedy evaporation.)

Commercially manufactured perfumes often contain animal scents as fixatives. In natural cosmetics, we can use as fixatives certain fragrances that keep up to a week. A plant oil (jojoba oil) can be used as a natural fixative instead of alcohol.

The perfumes that you can buy contain up to 20% fragrance. *Eau de perfume* has up to 15%, *eau de toilette* up to 5%, and eau de cologne up to 3%. The classical perfumes can be divided into the following groups:

- fresh, stimulating perfumes containing gardenia, violet, lilac, tuberose, etc.
- refreshing, nonaphrodisiac eaux de cologne, with lemon, orange, ginger, sage, spike lavender, thyme, verbena, bergamot, etc.
- stimulating, aphrodisiac perfumes featuring oak moss, musk, amber, tonka, sandalwood, patchouli, and jasmine—a euphoric flower bouquet with a great variety of blossom fragrances and a fresh top scent
- slightly aphrodisiac and stimulating perfumes without euphoric fragrances, made with carrot seed
- purely euphoric perfumes with rose, tuberose, jasmine, clary sage, ylang-ylang, benzoin, etc.
- soothing perfumes containing lavender, petitgrain, rosewood, bergamot, etc.

Creating Individualized Natural Perfumes

It is truly a pleasure to make your own perfume by selecting and mixing the oils. However, certain factors must be taken into consideration. Perfumes are composed of various fragrances. Like notes in a musical composition, some scents "play" a larger role, while others are "heard" only briefly; still others are placed in the middle, where they can determine the rhythm for a long time. In the language of perfume composition, there is a top scent composed of oils with a short-lived fragrance or those with a less intense fragrance. In between is the medium scent, containing fragrances that have medium evaporation time or are of average intensity. They link the top scent with the basic fragrance, the slow evaporating, heavy scents which are perceived the longest.

The secret of a perfect mixture lies in the consideration of scent intensities and the amount of individual oils. You would not perceive a mixture of 1 drop of Roman chamomile and 1 drop of lavender as a balanced composition of the two fragrances, since chamomile clearly has a stronger scent intensity: a single drop is equivalent in scent intensity to 6 drops of lavender!

The core of every composition is a blossom fragrance that determines the real character of the perfume. Ultimately you can only find out how a perfume smells on your skin by wearing it, because the perfume will mix with your own body scent. It is possible that a completely different fragrance may result.

I recommend that you first start with a small amount (⅓ oz.) of perfume. The little amber bottles for such small amounts can be obtained when you buy essential oils. Smell all of the oils and then choose the ones with the most pleasant fragrances. Put about 25–30 drops essential oils in the bottle. Shake the contents well.

If one or another ingredient smells too strongly, or if something seems to be missing, then you can attempt to balance out the mixture. Otherwise, add ⅓ oz. of jojoba oil, close the bottle, and shake the contents again. When you check the mixture, stay with your initial impression. Too much smelling can confuse an inexperienced nose.

Now keep the bottle closed for two weeks in order to allow the scents time to merge. After that time, you can examine the results of your first personalized perfume. If the scent has become too strong, dilute it with jojoba oil. The creation of an eau de toilette without alcohol is similar to the face lotion produced with flower water and essential oils (see page 98).

The tables in the Appendix provide basic information about fragrance characteristics, intensities, and evaporation values. Some oils are also listed that are not used in natural cosmetics but can be valuable in making perfume.

Recipes for Natural Perfumes

The following sample mixtures, meant to guide your first steps into the fragrant world of perfume-making, are all based on ⅓ oz. of jojoba oil. The amounts given are in drops.

Woody

15 cedarwood
5 sandalwood
5 rosewood
2 lemongrass

Sweet

4 neroli
4 rose
4 rosewood
4 cedarwood

Sweet, slightly aphrodisiac

4 jasmine
4 ylang-ylang
8 rosewood
1 vanilla
4 neroli

Refreshing, not aphrodisiac

10 bergamot
5 melissa
10 petitgrain
5 verbena

Heavy, exotic, aphrodisiac

10 patchouli
8 frankincense
6 ylang-ylang
4 jasmine

Strong, manly, aphrodisiac

15 sandalwood
5 carrot seed
3 ylang-ylang
1 clove

Very aphrodisiac

10 carrot seed
10 patchouli
5 ylang-ylang
5 cypress

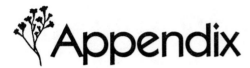

Appendix

Characteristic Fragrances of Essential Oils

Amber: aphrodisiac, flowery, musk-like, slightly sweet
Angelica root: earthy, slightly musk-like, peppery, aromatic
Anise: sweet, herbal, lively
Basil: penetrating, sweet, spicy, fresh, anise-like
Benzoin: sweet, balsamy, warm
Bergamot: fresh, clear, fruity-sweet
Cajeput: eucalyptus-like, intensely herbal
Camphor: medicinal
Caraway: strongly spicy
Cardamom: spicy, aromatic, balsamy-flowery
Carrot seed: woodsy-earthy
Cassia (Chin. cinnamon oil): intensely spicy, cinnamon-like
Cassie: spicy-flowery
Cedarwood: harmonious, soft wood fragrance, sweet-and-sour
Chamomile, blue: very sweet, herbal
Chamomile, Roman: fresh, sweet, herbal, tea-like

Cinnamon bark: strong, warm, spicy-sweet
Cinnamon leaves: warm, spicy, clove-like
Citronella (Java): slightly sweet, woodsy-flowery, rosy
Clary sage: light, slightly hay-like, spicy, similar to bergamot
Clove, flowers and leaves: strong, warm, spicy-sweet
Coriander: spicy, aromatic
Cypress: fresh, spicy, lemony-fruity
Eucalyptus citriodora: rosy, citronella-like
Eucalyptus globulus: camphor-like
Fennel: warm
Frankincense/Olibanum: balsamy, spicy, lemony
Geranium: leafy, rosy, minty-fruity
Ginger: spicy-woodsy, warm
Grapefruit: light, fresh, bitter
Hyacinth: intensively sweet, leafy, flowery, euphoric
Hyssop: sweet, spicy, camphor-like, woody-warm
Immortelle: honey-like, fruity, sweet, smells like tea and
    chamomile
Jasmine: honey-sweet, intensively flowery
Juniper: strong, herbal, scent of pine needles and gin
Lavender: sweet, balsamy, flowery
Lemon: fresh, bright
Lemongrass: fresh, similar to lemon and verbena, slightly bitter
Limette/Lime: intensive, sparkling-sweet, lemony
Marjoram: typical scent of the kitchen herb
Melissa: light, sparkling, minty-fruity
Mimosa: straw-like
Musk (Ambretta): aphrodisiac, musky, sweet-woody
Myrrh: warm, slightly spicy-sweet, balsamy, fine
Myrtle: spicy, hint of camphor and eucalyptus
Narcissus: earthy, straw-like, spicy
Neroli: sweet, spicy-bitter
Niaouli: light, fresh, eucalyptus-like
Nutmeg: light, typical smell of nutmeg spice
Oak moss: earthy, mossy, leather-like
Onion: penetrating, acrid

Orange, sweet: bright, fruity, clear, sweet

Oregano: spicy, tart-bitter, thyme-like, smells like the kitchen herb

Parsley seed: warm, spicy-herbal, smells like the kitchen herb

Patchouli: strongly woody-balsamy-sweet, woodsy, earthy

Pennyroyal: light, fresh, like camphor and mint

Pepper (black): warm, spicy, herbal, like the spice

Peppermint: minty-fresh, grass-like, balsamy-sweet

Petitgrain: weakly sweet, woodsy-flowery, similar to neroli

Pine and pine needle: tart, spicy, fresh

Rose: (depends on flower type) sweet, rosy

Rosewood: flowery, slightly rosy, spicy-sweet

Sage: strong, fresh-spicy, herbal, medicinal

Sandalwood: balsamy-sweet, velvety-warm

Savory: fresh, herb-like, medicinal, thyme-like

Tangerine: bright, fresh, typical fruit fragrance

Tarragon: anise-like, strong, spicy, celery-like

Tea tree: strong, camphor-like, herbal

Thuja: fresh, camphor-like, spicy

Thyme: strong, herbal-sweet, slightly medicinal

Tuberose: heavy, honey-like, sweet, flowery, euphoric

Vanilla extract: sweet, warm, balsamy

Verbena: fresh, fruity, citrus-like

Vetiver: heavy, woodsy-earthy, sweet-and-sour, woody-balsamy

Violet: leafy, herbal, peppery

Ylang-ylang: narcotic-sweet, strong, jasminey

Note: Not all of the essential oils smell like the flowers, herbs, or plants from which they are extracted.

Fragrance Types

Flowery scents
- bergamot
- cassie
- citronella
- geranium
- jasmine
- lavender
- neroli
- petitgrain
- rose
- rosewood
- tuberose
- violet
- ylang-ylang

Earthy scents
- angelica root
- carrot seed
- narcissus
- oak moss
- patchouli
- vetiver

Woodsy, mossy, leafy scents
- carrot seed
- cedarwood
- geranium
- hyacinth
- oak moss
- patchouli
- pine
- violet
- vetiver

Fresh scents
- basil
- bergamot
- citronella
- cypress
- eucalyptus
- grapefruit
- lemon
- lemongrass
- limette/lime
- melissa
- peppermint
- pine
- sage
- savory
- thuja
- verbena

Herbal scents
- anise
- chamomile, Roman
- juniper
- marjoram
- oregano
- parsley
- pepper
- sage
- savory
- thyme

Honey scents
- honey
- immortelle
- jasmine
- tuberose

Warm scents
- bensoin
- cinnamon
- clove
- fennel
- frankincense
- myrrh
- orange
- parsley
- pepper
- sandalwood
- vanilla

Sweet scents
- anise
- basil
- bergamot
- benzoin
- chamomile, blue
- chamomile, Roman
- cinnamon bark
- citronella
- clove blossom
- hyssop
- honey

Sweet scents (continued)
immortelle
jasmine
lavender
limette/lime
myrrh
neroli
orange
patchouli
petitgrain
rose
rosewood
sandalwood
savory
tangerine
tuberose
vanilla
ylang-ylang

Sweet and heavy scents
amber
bensoin
cinnamon bark
jasmine
musk
neroli
parchouli
rose
vanilla
vetiver
ylang-ylang

Narcotic scents
hyacinth
rose
tuberose
ylang-ylang

Rose-like scents
citronella
eucalyptus
   citriodora
rose geranium
rose
rosewood

Mossy, woody,
leathery, masculine
scents
cedarwood
clove
hyssop
nutmeg
oak moss
patchouli
sandalwood
vetiver

Musky scents
amber
angelica root

Aphrodisiac scents
cardamon
cinnamon
clary sage
jasmine
musk
neroli
patchouli
rose
sandalwood
vanilla
ylang-ylang

Erotic scents
amber
carrot seed
cypress
frankincense
geranium
musk
myrrh

Relaxing scents
basil
bergamot
cedarwood
chamomile,
   Roman
clary sage
fennel
frankincense
geranium
jasmine
lavender
marjoram
melissa
myrrh
neroli
orange
patchouli
rose
rosewood
sandalwood
ylang-ylang

Stimulating scents
camphor
cardamom
cinnamon

Stimulating scents
(continued)
  clary sage
  clove
  coriander
  eucalyptus
  ginger
  juniper

peppermint
rosemary
thyme
verbena

Euphoric scents
  clary sage
  clove

grapefruit
jasmine
neroli
orange
rose
ylang-ylang

Fragrance Intensity
(insofar as these have been measured and are known)

Light	*Medium*	*Strong*
bergamot	amber	chamomile, blue
camphor	anise	clove
cedarwood	basil	eucalyptus
cinnamon	cajeput	frankincense
clove	camphor	garlic
cypress	carrot seed	hyacinth
fennel	chamomile, Roman	jasmine
grapefruit	citronella	mimosa
juniper	clary sage	neroli
lemon	fennel	peppermint
marjoram	geranium	vanilla
melissa	honey	violet
myrrh	lavender	ylang-ylang
nutmeg	lemongrass	
pennyroyal	niaouli	
petitgrain	oak moss	
pine	orange	
tangerine	patchouli	
tea tree	rosewood	
verbena	sage	
	sandalwood	
	thyme	
	verbena	

Degree of Volatility
(insofar as these have been measured and are known)

Approximate values: scent disappears in the air at normal room temperature within one day for fast oils, after two days for medium oils, after one week for slow oils.

Fast (top note)	Medium (top note)	Slow (base note)
bergamot	anise	benzoin
chamomile, blue	basil	cedarwood
chamomile, Roman	clove	clary sage
eucalyptus	cypress	frankincense
grapefruit	fennel	geranium
juniper	grapefruit	ginger
lemon	hyssop	jasmine
marjoram	lavender	myrrh
pennyroyal	niaouli	neroli
rosemary	nutmeg	patchouli
rosewood	orange	rose
	pepper	sandalwood
	peppermint	vanilla
	petitgrain	ylang-ylang
	pine	
	sage	
	tangerine	
	thyme	
	verbena	

Table of Quantities for the Use of Essential Oils

20 drops essential oils is equivalent to about 1 gram = 0.0353 ounce.

A 1% dilution of 2 (4) ounce of vegetable oil or emulsion is equivalent to about 20 (40) drops essential oils.

A 3% dilution of 2 (4) ounces ofvegetable oil or emulsion is equivalent to about 60 (120) drops essential oils:

Skin care oils have a 1–2 % dilution. Healing oils have a 3% dilution.

For aromatic skin care baths, use 6–15 drops essential oils.

For facial compresses and steam baths, use a maximum of 10 drops essential oils in 2 pints of water.

For a skin toner, use up to a maximum of 5 drops essential oils in 4 ounces of water.

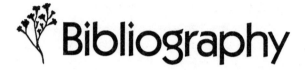

Bibliography

Davis, Patricia. *Aromatherapy, an A–Z*. Walden, Essex: C.W. Daniel, 1988. An extensive handbook on all of the symptoms and essential oils; based on average knowledge of medicine.

Hampton, Aubrey. *Natural Organic Hair and Skin Care*. Tampa, Fla.: Organica Press, 1987. Includes a very complete guide to natural and synthetic chemicals in cosmetics.

Keller, Erich. *The Complete Home Guide to Aromatherapy*. Tiburon, Calif.: H. J. Kramer, 1991. Contains a description of the 77 most important oils; an easy introduction to the methods of aromatherapy and the use of essential oils.

Tisserand, Robert B. *The Art of Aromatherapy*. Rochester, Vt.: Healing Arts Press, 1977. A classic text on aromatherapy and essential oils.

Winter, Ruth. *A Consumer's Dictionary of Cosmetic Ingredients*. New York: Crown Publishers, 1984. Alphabetical listing of all natural and synthetic cosmetic ingredients. Highly recommended.

Suppliers of Essential Oils

Aroma Vera
3384 South Robertson Place
Los Angeles, CA 90034
(213) 280-0407
essential oils

Original Swiss Aromatics
PO Box 606
San Rafael, CA 94915
(415) 459-3998
essential oils

Santa Fe Fragrance Inc.
PO Box 282
Santa Fe, NM 87504
(505) 473-1717
botanical essential oils, bulk available, send SASE for price list

Tiferet Intl.
210 Crest Drive
Eugene, OR 97405
(503) 344-7019
essential oils

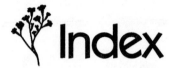 Index